What people are saying about

108 Steps to God

Some books are like textbooks for life – filled with such nuggets of wisdom and invaluable advice that you highlight favorite sentences to refer back to for guidance, inspiration and hope. This is one of those books; an intensely personal account of Anne-Marie Newland's experiences and the myriad lessons she has learned. Candid, witty and enlightening, Anne-Marie doesn't pretend to have all the answers to life's mysteries, but she is generous, insightful and sincere about the revelations she has gained through her magical yoga practice.

This is a book everyone can benefit from. It speaks to me as a Buddhist, a working woman and as a mother. Some people have an ability to touch others profoundly with their writing because they're so scrupulously honest with themselves. Anne-Marie is blessed with this gift – she is a true Teacher.

Julie Peasgood, TV & stage actress and Buddhist

108 Steps to God

Dealing with God's Jokes

108 Steps to God

Dealing with God's Jokes

Anne-Marie Newland

BOOKS

Winchester, UK
Washington, USA

First published by O-Books, 2019
O-Books is an imprint of John Hunt Publishing Ltd., 3 East St., Alresford,
Hampshire SO24 9EE, UK
office1@jhpbooks.net
www.johnhuntpublishing.com

For distributor details and how to order please visit the 'Ordering' section on our website.

Text copyright: Anne-Marie Newland 2018

ISBN: 978 1 78535 666 7
978 1 78535 667 4 (ebook)
Library of Congress Control Number: 2017932886

A CIP catalogue record for this book is available from the British Library.

Design: Stuart Davies

Printed and bound by CPI Group (UK) Ltd, Croydon, CR0 4YY, UK

We operate a distinctive and ethical publishing philosophy in
all areas of our business, from our global network of authors to
production and worldwide distribution.

Contents

Other books by Anne-Marie Newland:
Sun Power Yoga SHALA
Published 2015 by Sun Power Publishing

This book is dedicated to my four children
who regularly help me out of the gutter!

Acknowledgments

The cornerstones, Jamie, Melissa, Liam Newland and Talitha Hepple-Newland.

My nieces and nephews, Nathan, Joseph, Satya-Sara and Theresa Khachik.

My sister Shereen and brothers Ramzy and Samir.

Cathlene Kidston-Fitt, who worked with me on this book and puts up with my amateur dramatics.

And a special thank you to everybody who has ever given me a hard time.

Preface

This book is about God's Jokes. You know, the ones the Divine laughs at while you pick yourself up out of the gutter again. This is my personal view of those Jokes, how I dealt with them and what made me get up and carry on. I include my family as well as my work and I am certain some of these dark tales will resonate with you.

● ● ●

God never sends suffering. Never. It is never 'God's will' that we should suffer. God would like us not to suffer. But since the world brings suffering, and since God refuses to use His almighty power and treat us as foolish children, He aligns Himself with us, goes into Auschwitz with us, is devastated by 9/11 with us, and draws us with Him through it all into fulfillment. This is a high price to pay for our human freedom, but it is worth it. To be mere automatons for whom God arranges the world to cause us no suffering would mean we never have a Self. We could not make choices.

-*Sister Wendy Beckett*

Foreword

If, of thy mortal goods, thou art bereft,
And from thy slender store two loaves alone to thee are
left,
Sell one and from the dole,
Buy Hyacinths to feed the soul.
-Muslih-uddin Sadi, 13th Century Persian Poet

OM

When Anne-Marie asked me to write a forward for her new book, I was flattered, touched - and just a bit puzzled as to what to write. So, I thought I'd start with an offering of my favorite poem.

Anne-Marie warned me in advance that her book was 'unusual' - and knowing Anne-Marie, I had no doubt that it would be. She said that it dealt with some pretty radical concepts: motherhood, divorce, struggles, etc.

I have known Anne-Marie since 1983 when she came to work with Swami Vishnu Devananda in London, when she was a serious fashionista and rockette! I know that she has faced all the obstacles that she speaks about in her book - not only confronted them, but accepted the challenges with a smile. She has let her challenges make her stronger - and she has always passed that strength on to her students.

The real radicalness of Anne-Marie's book is that it is full of suggestions that could cause a real inner foment. Reading them reminded me of the title of a book by the Indian philosopher J. Krishnamurti *The Only Revolution* - he was referring to meditation.

The suggestions of this book ask us to let go of many of our pet preconceptions and to take responsibility for our own lives. While presenting them in a painless way, Anne-Marie is inviting us to overthrow our attachments to our weaknesses. Her suggestions are in keeping with those of Krishna in the Bhagavad Gita (6.23) when he defines Yoga as the cutting of the connection to pain.

Sometimes when I'm teaching philosophy to yoga teachers, I hear a student mention the '8-steps of yoga'. I always stop her to clarify this common misnomer of the Sanskrit word *anga*. It would be more correct to render the word as 'limb' or 'part'. I'm mentioning this, not to be pedantic, but because as I was reading Anne-Marie's impassioned book, I realized that her 108 steps are not actually steps, because steps are things that you climb in a particular order – and hopefully take one at a time.

In reality, Anne-Marie has provided us with 108 viable paths. You can take them in any order – or just take one and use it as an inspiration for your continued practice.

In my forty years of teaching yoga and meditation, I've found that people want someone to take away their bad habits, but really all they need to do is give them up. They wish for patience, but don't realize that it comes as the result of tribulations. They dream of happiness, but the decision to be happy is up to them.

My hope is that you will choose at least one of Anne-Marie's dynamic suggestions – and really use it! If you do, I'm sure that you will find that you have arrived at a more peaceful and joyful life.

With prayers and best wishes.

Swami Saradananda

●————— ● ● ● —————●

Swami Saradananda is an internationally renowned yoga and meditation teacher who has inspired thousands of people to practice.

For 26 years, she worked with the International Sivananda Yoga Vedanta Centers and directed their facilities in New York, London, New Delhi and the Himalayas. After an extended period of personal practice in the Himalayas in 2001, she was 'author in residence' at the Peacemaker Community in Western Massachusetts, and she then went on to direct yoga and meditation retreat Haus Yoga Vidya, just outside of Cologne, Germany.

Swami Saradananda teaches yoga worldwide, leads pilgrimages to India and writes extensively.

She is also a trustee of the Ganga Prem Hospice, a charity that is seeking to build a cancer hospice in Rishikesh, North India.

A Note from the Author

The Courage to Break Out

I was born in Kirkuk, Iraq, in 1955. My Father was Iraqi, and his parents, my grandparents, were Armenian. My Mother was English, with Scottish and Portuguese roots. I was born into the Syrian Orthodox faith and am comfortable with both my faith and my Yoga Philosophy. I am familiar with incense, candles and chanting; I heard them each day when I went to church with my Grandmother in Baghdad. I used to feel safe kneeling at her side, watching as those around us became silent, still and luminescent, with what I now know is the Wisdom and Light of Faith.

I was exiled with my family in 1960, leaving behind my Father: a political prisoner of the despotic regime in power at the time, still known as the Baath party of the late Saddam Hussein.

My life has been blessed with four children, has been brutal, exotic, challenging, frightening, overwhelming, deeply passionate and exhilarating. I have done things people only dream about and experienced things people would hope never to experience, even in their worst nightmares.

'Serious' Yoga came into my life as an epiphany in 1983 after practicing Hatha Yoga without the Spiritual parts that make Yoga what it is: the Mind, the Body and the Breath.

The first yoga class I attended was with my late Mother in 1972. She had been practicing for some time, starting at home by watching the ground breaking Lynn Marshall in an all-in-one lycra body suit, on television. We still have a long-playing LP with Lynn talking through the basics of a Yoga practice, and I'm sure I still have my Mother's purple lycra leotard, too!

I lived at a boarding school in Tring back then, having

been given a scholarship to study ballet. While I was home in Leicester, my Mother suggested I try her yoga class to keep supple during the long holidays. We went along to the YMCA and I placed myself in the shadows to keep out of view of the teacher. As a ballet dancer I was very flexible and teachers loved to use me as an example. I hated that so I slunk into the darkest recess.

Well, the experience of that first yoga class almost put me off for life! Not only were the women wearing lycra all-in-ones but so were the men! Their beer bellies thrust forward like peacocks. And no one warned me about how noisy it could be; I thought Yoga was quiet and calming!

My Mother lay down near me on a towel – no yoga mats in those days. As the teacher took us through the basics, the women and men were breaking wind randomly, and with pride and vigor, all around the class! I was horrified. I was only sixteen for heaven's sake and breaking wind was something to be avoided at all cost. I looked at my Mother in shock and disapproval.

Putting on her best Queen Elizabeth accent, Mom said, "Better out than in!"

That was the last Yoga I did until 1976 and even then I entered the class with trepidation!

Many years have passed since then and I realize now that I felt similar to lots of people who think Yoga is for the middle-aged and is slow, consists mostly of lying around and is some sort of weird cult or is only for celebrities, plus, you have to be a contortionist in order to do it! The good news is, things have changed dramatically. Yoga is out of the closet and in the mainstream.

Like anything that achieves celebrity status, fame can also mean a loss of something, and for me this loss was in the areas of integrity, knowledge, vocation, true meaning and depth, and as a path for the spiritual aspirant. These were the metaphorical 'babies' thrown out, together with the 'OM' mantra, in the bath water. This is where I feel so privileged to know that the training I had and my introduction to Yoga was both authentic and old school.

I am old school; there is no doubt about it. I still believe in teachers. I believe the student needs commitment and discipline from that teacher. I don't mean corporal punishment, but to learn self-discipline. Yoga is a step toward that self-discipline. There is an expression that says that the student searches for the teacher and that the teacher will arrive when the time is right.

For myself, that is a profound statement and one that is nothing but a truth.

In 1976 I was going through one of the most difficult and emotionally challenging times of my life thus far. It was the summer of the 1976 heat wave. People were on the streets trying to keep cool, hoses were out to keep the children's temperature down and it was such fun. London was buzzing with an outdoor life a long time before there were street cafes to go to.

I was in love and in pain. By 1977 I had no money, nowhere to live, a family who were very poor and no one who could help. I had troubles I could not share with anyone. I walked over to the library in Stoke Newington. Since childhood I had found solace in books and in the silence of the buildings. Books jumped out at me. The first time I remember this happening, I was nine years old and in my local library. That time it was a text that would determine how I looked after my skin, my body, and would help me develop my own perception of beauty.

This day was no different. I never seemed to know exactly how or when, but suddenly, with little recollection, I had a book in my hands. I turned it over. It was an unfamiliar title, austere and serious: *Hatha Yoga* by T. Bernard. Of course, this little book, with sepia pictures of Bernard in what seemed impossible shapes, is now recognized as a torch, lighting the way for the Western Yogi and has been reprinted. I would like to apologize to Islington Library for never returning their copy on the 17th May 1977 when it was due back!

That book saved me that summer. No matter the drama happening in my personal life, I got up each day to practice these strange shapes, called *Asana*, with my body. They were vaguely reminiscent of the shapes my Mother's class had adopted, but the energy and the intent behind them were far more powerful. I read about meditation, breathing and mental focus. It was this that had been the missing key. I sought out a local yoga class and found an Iyengar one running at the local adult education center. That teacher was Maxine Tobias. She was, and still is, an exponent of Iyengar strength, technique and severe alignment. I enjoyed the classes and remembered that a man called Iyengar had been in the UK in 1976, taking workshops, and I read many years later that Eric Schiffmann was there and had met with a punch on the chin from Iyengar when he dropped his chin while in warrior pose! Traditional Yoga can be very harsh. The West has tempered this harshness, as most people find it difficult to deal with, but as a ballet dancer this strict discipline was normal to me.

I was used to being physically abused as a ballet dancer, and the nature of my Iyengar classes were sometimes similar to the stress I felt then—strict alignment and super postures—but my heart was not in it. My body was a piece of art, a sculpture that had been worked on since I was six years old. It didn't feel as though it was mine. It was a tool and instrument but I didn't exist within it. Yoga began to lose its hold on me and I was disappointed but wasn't sure why. Why was it that the practice didn't hold me, not like the book I had read? What was missing? Had I still not understood what Yoga was?

After a career as a ballet and contemporary dancer, taught by Arlene Philips, Richard Branson (Virgin Music) gave me my first job as a choreographer for Vangelis, of 'Chariots of Fire' fame, at his very first UK concert at the Albert Hall in London. My choreography included the dancers having to dance and play the timpani, which is where my passion for drumming began. I then had a brief spell as a punk drummer with Toyah Willcox's band and featured in the cult film 'Jubilee' by Derek Jarman. I supported the Clash in 1978, after which I bought a boutique and became a fashion designer for the stars and a make-up artist for a video company. Then I had an epiphany, and my rock and roll life ended right there, forever, in May 1983.

I received a series of divine messages that led me to a place in my life I was scared of. I was leaving my old, familiar life of 'sex, drugs and rock 'n' roll' behind me and taking a leap into a life of Spirituality. The unknown is always terrifying, but I felt it was the right path for me. I was led to the Sivananda Yoga Centre in Notting Hill. I took my first class. My teacher became my husband within three months and Swami Vishnu married us. It was that easy. I've never looked back, not ever. Being taught by Swamiji was such a privilege. I was at the right place at the right time. Swamiji lived in Canada most of the time but travelled as much as he could to his centers and ashrams. He was younger than you might imagine him to be, and a striking figure in his orange robes and bare feet. He had a smile and a cheeky laugh that was easy to feel at ease with. He was also very strict and, as is the tradition of revered teachers in India, he demanded respect.

This aspect of tradition is where I'm old school. In the past, teachers were automatically given respect. Subsequent generations seem to have questioned this, expecting teachers to earn their respect before they will give it. In fact, teachers should always be given respect, until they lose it, not the other way around. I would go further and say we ALL deserve respect first, with no conditions, until we demonstrate otherwise. Only then do we have to work, hard, to earn it back.

When I decided to let my other life go and to follow this real path and life, I had many lessons to learn. I was a spitfire, a defiant young person who was not afraid to have a voice. I stood up for others if they could not, or would not, stand up for themselves. I hated injustice, bullying and prejudice. What I had to learn from my Spiritual life was that at times one must not ask questions or expect any answers.

I travelled out to Canada with Swamiji's insulin; he was a diabetic and people always say, "How come? Why didn't he look after himself?" A spiritual practice can be a paradox. Not eating *Tamasic* food, like meat, keeps the blood steady and the mind free of fear, but eating *Satvic* foods, like sugar, is bad for the body, yet nice for the mind, and sitting for meditation for hours or days as the monks do is not great for your joints, spine, or knees but it is good for the soul!

I started my training the wrong way round. I went to Canada to follow my husband, who was building a Shiva fountain at the Sivananda HQ in the Laurentien Mountains. While I was there I joined in a teacher-training course as a guest, after which I decided I should officially sign up for a course I wanted to do in India.

Listening to Swami Vishnu's lectures (*Satsang*) each evening, in his small, modest home (*shala*) was inspiring. He was funny and his stories down-to-earth and easy to understand. They expressed compassion for ourselves, for others and for the world. His Guru was Swami Sivananda of Rishikesh, who brought to the West a Yoga that was integrated: the breath, the poses, the diet, the meditation and the positive thinking. For me, his Yoga has stayed true to its roots but has been allowed to grow for the West in a way that has been adopted by all backgrounds, faiths and cultures. He was a medical doctor and, as a functional anatomist, I see a good understanding of the inner body and inner mind in his writing and teachings. He was practical, and this is the part I make sure is kept alive in my teachings.

My Mother practiced Iyengar Yoga in her later life. She carried on with the practice until she could no longer walk because of cancer, bless her. What a legacy she left me. She believed that knowledge was the greatest teacher and always encouraged me to never rest in the pursuit of wisdom.

I have studied Astanga Vinyasa Yoga with some of the great teachers. It fed the dancer in me and I know that the blend of threads I learned from Maxine Tobias's Iyengar class, and the grace I learned with Swami Vishnu, created the Yoga I teach today. I am a mother, a single mother, a mentor, a disciplinarian, a Karma Yogi, a maverick, a pain in the bottom (often) but I can stand up and say I am a pioneer and was never too afraid to break the rules. Yoga, like everything, needs its traditional roots, but also needs to grow and change. This way we allow more room for those who were once excluded by those who felt Yoga was only for the right caste or class. I'm an anarchist in that case! I believe we are all God's children, and, no matter what your religion or faith, Yoga speaks the same familiar language of compassion: a prayer expressed through the body, mind and breath.

— • • • —

I have found my purpose; I am a teacher.
I had the courage to break out and dance my own dance.
To be an authentic teacher we need more than technique, knowledge or practice.
"We need the Eye, the Hand and the Heart."

— • • • —

About This Book

This series of 108 steps to God are truths that I have come to understand and use to get me through my life in 'Sunshine'. Some days and years are harder than others but if we can find a point to focus on and steadfastly travel our road with an inner durability and hope, then that is all we can ask of ourselves.

It occurred to me that it might be useful to others to note that hardship, joy, love and loss are universal and that the ways in which we deal with them are myriad and possibly not so universal! You can use this book as you wish. You may like to read each entry in its order, which is my preference. Or you may like to use the guidance of inspiration, questions, or ask the Divine to open the book on a random page. Use this book, but also put into practice things you want to work on or experience. The main purpose is to feel it is worthwhile and useful to see the lightness in some of God's Jokes!

Why 108 Steps?

108 represents the 108 beads on the Mala, the string of beads by which we practice Japa meditation. The Sanskrit word *japa* is derived from the root *jap-*, meaning, 'to utter in a low voice, repeat internally, mutter'. Japa meditation is the repeating of a mantra, the sacred sound of the Universe, the first sound. The Earth in orbit makes the sound 'OM' for instance, pronounced A-U-M. This is repeated silently in the mind as we pass each bead through our finger and thumb on a breath: inhale, OM, pass a bead, exhale, OM, and pass a bead. The use of the Mala beads is a tool to aid the focus and application of the mind's absorption in this practice.

Mālā, in its grossest translation, means 'garland' and its deepest meaning is 'to cleanse of negativity'. Mala beads help to keep the mind focused on the work of meditating and clear it of any unrelated thoughts. A Mala looks very much like a Rosary or the worry beads that Arabs use to keep the mind clear. There is an additional bead (Guru bead, Meru bead, Root bead) usually with a small tassel attached, which measures each round. This is the 109th bead, not the 108th. Ideally, you should try to complete three Malas (rounds).

You can read about many different ways to try Japa meditation with the Mala beads, so where and how to start?

It is already pretty challenging getting down to meditating in the first place, and while I do believe in keeping some traditions, not if it stops people trying the Mala beads! We live in a modern society and I'm traditional, yet flexible in my teaching of these complex ways because I want this often dry method to be useful and not a hindrance to personal spiritual development.

Things change all the time, even in ancient arts, so I always tell my students, "Do what feels good and comfortable, as it will help you to settle into meditating without worrying about a right or wrong way." My interpretation of Swami Vishnu's philosophies is, why make things difficult when often people need to feel normal doing spiritual stuff, not elitist, alienated or plain stupid.

Traditionally, you rest the Mala beads on your middle or ring finger, not your index finger. The index finger is known as 'the finger of Indignation', used when people are telling someone off or being angry, and shouldn't touch the Mala beads.

Having said that, if you want to use the index finger, then it's about feeling comfortable enough to try. Left handed people find it easier to use the index finger...as one must not use the left hand due to the Indian tradition of using the left hand for cleaning the bottom and the right for food.

So, sit with the beads in the right hand, with the root bead between your preferred finger and thumb.

Let the beads rest where feels comfortable, with the hand on the end of the knee.

Some traditionalists will say that the beads should not hang below the navel and shouldn't touch the floor, however it is very uncomfortable trying to keep them above the navel, especially for beginners, and I like the idea of the beads resting on the floor, symbolizing the connection to Earth (physical) and the aspiration of the mind to connect to the divine (Heaven), with the person as the connection between the two.

Each bead passes between your finger and thumb. As you pass each bead through your fingers, as well as the breath, try repeating in your mind the mantra 'OM'.

When you reach the 108th bead, if you wish to continue your meditation and complete another round, traditionally, you turn the Mala beads in your hand and go back the other way, not passing the root bead through your fingers. Swamiji taught me how to use the beads many moons ago, and he never mentioned not crossing the root bead, also it is very hard not to do when you are a novice! So, if you find it easier, allow the root bead to pass through your fingers and complete another round in the same direction as before.

All these methods and simple tools are to aid us, like incense or candles help us associate with mindfulness, focus and stillness by the scent or the light they produce.

• —————— • • • —————— •

One bead is an in-breath and the next bead the out-breath. Each bead is a mantra or OM, the simplest and most potent of sounds.
These mantras are silently repeated and synchronized with the breath until a magnetic and rhythmic pulse is created through your whole body, connecting beautifully and seamlessly with the mind.

———— • • • ————

The *slokas* (Sanskrit verse) are divided into three parts, *Satva*, *Rajas* and *Tamas*. These are the three Gunas or personalities of God, life and man, together with everything on our Earth and beyond. They also reflect the three faces of God: Brahma the Creator, Vishnu the Preserver and Shiva the destroyer, as explained in Hindu texts.

Satva: Birth, purity, innocence, new life, sweetness. The early morning (dawn) has these personalities, as do people and especially children.

Rajas: Action, growth, fire, work, achievement, sunshine and Karma Yoga. The daytime has these qualities.

Tamas: Death, inertia, endings. The evening has this personality as the sun lowers and we move into darkness.

You may wish to simply watch the breath, in on one bead, out on the next. What could be more powerful than connecting to breath? Nothing, as breath is life. The ancient sages said that life couldn't be measured by time but by the breath, the less breaths the more time. Medically we know this to be true. High blood pressure and stress can produce fast breathing, so it can be seen as spending breaths rather than experiencing them.

One of my students, a GP, who was training with me a few years ago, asked me, while I was teaching her group about the Mala beads and meditation, why 108 beads? I explained that in Yoga philosophy the number 108 has significance for many reasons.

- The numbers 9 and 12 both have spiritual significance: 9 x 12 = 108.
- The diameter of the Sun is 108 times the diameter of the Earth. The distance from the Sun to the Earth is 108 times the diameter of the Sun.
- The average distance of the Moon from the Earth is 108

times the diameter of the Moon.

- 108 is a Harshad number, meaning it is a number divisible by the sum of its digits (*Harshad* is Sanskrit for 'great joy').
- The individual numbers, 1, 0, 8 represent one thing, nothing and everything.

I suggest you consider that there are also 108 reasons!

•——————— • • • ———————•

"Just think of the Mala beads as 108 steps to God," I said. "Anne-Marie! That's a title for a book!"

•——————— • • • ———————•

I was taught very early on in my own spiritual quest that the most important road to Yoga was meditation, Raja Yoga, The Royal Road, and the Mala beads are an intricate part of that first journey. This meant little to me at the time. Since 1984 my progress has been interestingly slow. What I have learned is that there are many paths in Yoga and that the best to start with is Hatha Yoga, the physical aspects of this ancient discipline.

Now I know that people who practice Hatha Yoga don't always know that Hatha is a 'path' not a style of Yoga. There are eight limbs of Yoga[1] and one is Asana, which is the physical aspect of Yoga, as in poses. Hatha Yoga is the deeper layers within the physical aspect of Yoga[2]. This is a great place to begin, as we are inside a vehicle called the body. In the grossest term, our soul or spirit is a fragment of the divine and is carried by way of this vehicle. Hatha, in its simplest form, actually means 'effort'. It is an effort to make the body do what we want it to. As we become more advanced, I prefer to say more 'Mind-full' rather than 'Mind-less', the word Hatha shows its other complexities, such as Ha, 'Sun' and Tha, 'Moon'. The light and shade of this is amazing and, in the 21st century, is a totally relevant here-and-now philosophy. When I explain to any students that all the Asana practice (Hatha) they will do over years is simply to allow the body to sit comfortably so they can meditate...there is a look of confusion, shock and panic! Confusion because this is not what they signed up for, shock because they have signed up (and paid!) and panic because, deep down, they knew all along this was what they signed up for, and now they have to get on with it!

I can remember feeling exactly the same the first day I entered a small ashram in Notting Hill, back in 1983. I had heard a clear message (in my right ear) that I should "Practice Yoga seriously!" I had no idea that Yoga was serious. 'Seriously' meant I had to discover that it was not about practicing or performing beautifully executed postures, but that there was a philosophy, scriptures, paths and limbs, in short, a sacred structure which it became clear to me was very similar to my Christian Orthodox upbringing.

I made it to my first class at Notting Hill on the very day I had my epiphany, and I remember standing in the hall with my new life stretching out in front of me, and my other life disappearing behind me. I had arrived at a point I could no longer deny myself. I was scared and I could have changed my mind, but instead, I walked in. That day, my life changed forever, and the lives of many of my closest friends. We have all gone on to work in a deep and profound way across the world.

How lucky was I? How lucky were we all?

Endnotes

1 Patanjali's 8 Limbs of Yoga are Yama, Niyama, Asana, Pranayama, Pratyahara, Dharana, Dhyana and Samadhi.

2   The Hatha Yoga Pradipika is the greatest written authority on the physical aspects of Yoga. Anne-Marie's Book *Sun Power Yoga SHALA* covers this in detail.

The Root Bead

I am made up of my Mother's enigmatic, theatrical Englishness and of my Father's dry humor, harsh hand and ultimate sacrifices. I am not them but I recognize them in me. A potion made from ingredients from different sides of the world.

I love tea and cake and I love Arab coffee and Baklava.

I am made of the desert and I am flavored with grey fog and Michaelmas daisies.

My eyes reflect the skyline of Mosques and also the low sun of wintered Sunday mornings.

I am that I am.

● ● ●

1 The First Step is the Hardest

Try this, stand or sit with your eyes open, look out at the world as if your Soul is looking out, not you.

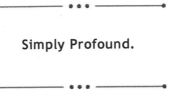

Simply Profound.

2 Find Your Way

My youngest daughter was 16 when she told me, very clearly, that Yoga had ruined her life because I was always doing something that included it! First lesson: remind yourself that you cannot try to live another's life or walk another's path. Stay on your own path because you want to and because it's about whom you are, no matter how others may feel about it!

3

We are all unique in every cell
If you do not strive to discover that uniqueness, something
*   has been lost forever*
Not just for you but for the Universe

4 Being 'On a Path' Seems like a Much Used Cliché

A cliché is something that everyone talks about. Therefore,

it stands to reason that someone else also experienced the thought you had. Therefore, 'The Path' must exist or we wouldn't mention it so often.

●—————— ● ● ● —————●

Clichés are much used truths.

●—————— ● ● ● —————●

5 Making a Start

I saw a small sign tacked onto a door in a Canadian Ashram. It said, 'Knock and you shall be answered'. This I knew to be of Christian doctrine, and I am ashamed to say that I so wanted to knock on that door and didn't have the courage. It's a pointless and deeply exhausting experience swimming against the tide when you are the only one who seems to be swimming.

●—————— ● ● ● —————●

At least knock and find out if it's the right door for you.

●—————— ● ● ● —————●

6 Once the Door has Opened

When you have crossed the threshold, it takes a lot of courage to sit down and listen. My first *Satsang*, 'meeting of like-minded people', consisted of a lecture on spiritual life, chanting in Sanskrit and prayers. I felt very hot and awkward. I looked around at the 'shiny, happy people holding hands' and thought,

'I am not going to throw myself into this 100 percent, just in case I need to run away out of that door'. I look at this now, many years later, and can truly align myself with these thoughts, but what if I hadn't stepped over the red line? Where would I be? Who would I be?

I tell my teachers, when they come though my doors, to get away from the wall, the place which is neither here nor there, and to commit.

— • • • —

Take your coat off and join the party.

— • • • —

7 Sit

What is Yoga anyway? It's a lot of people sitting down on their bottoms 'omming'. That is the most common answer given to me by lots of students and passers by. My answer is, "I wish," because if people sat down and 'ommed' then they would be too focused on themselves to give anyone else a hard time! Live your own life; don't try to force your lifestyle on others.

8 Open Your Eyes Wide and Take a Good Look Around You

Often we are only half awake. Sat between the Earth's reality and the Mind's fantasy we are not even aware of how to open our eyes. In Vedic philosophy there is the concept of *Maya*, 'illusion'. Maya is illustrated in stories as a female with a veil across her face. We only get an outline of her features and the rest we make up. How many times in your life have you thought you knew someone, something, a situation, only to find it was very different to your understanding. The veil dropped and you saw clearly. It can be a shock to find out you were so wrong, but also a great opportunity to learn from...if you have the courage.

9 Open Your Mouth Wide and Say Nothing but What is Needed

Taking the time to watch your words is another form of meditation. Slowing down the stream of thoughts that flow like a river over the waterfall allows space between the thought and the action. Think about the times you have said something in haste or anger and regretted it. Once the word and sound are released it is too late to bring them back. They are allowed to grow in strength and impact and the atmosphere they produce is tangible.

There is a story about the sandalwood tree - it takes many, many years to mature, and when the axe-man's blade cuts through its trunk, it releases its perfume. 'You could cut the air with a knife' is a cliché describing a bad atmosphere or bad feelings resulting from angry or ill-considered words, but speaking less and with mindfulness releases into the ether the mind perfume of that sandalwood tree: Love and Compassion.

10 Open Your Hands and See the Life You Have Been Living

Taking a look at the calluses on your hands tells you a little about your life. In past history, writers such as Dickens would describe a person's livelihood and profession by their hands. A land worker's rough, thick skin and the marks of physical labor told us they toiled every day. The white, slim, soft hands of the gentry showed they did no physical labor and were landowners. When I was first in India, training to be a Yoga teacher, I met many castes. After all the work of Mahatma Gandhi trying to rid India of the caste system, it still lives. The Swamis gave us all Karma Yoga duties (selfless service, working without reward, working for the sake of the action and not the result of that action) to perform while we trained. The Brahmins, the highest caste of scholars and religious families, were given the task of cleaning the toilets. This was usually left for the lower castes. During the course I had made friends with a young Brahmin boy, who confessed he had loved his job cleaning the toilets; it made him feel whole and purposeful. He also said that his mother would never let him do it when he returned home. I told him that he, not his mother, must walk his path. He laughed and said he would do his best!

11 Open Your Wallet and Give Your Last Hour

Charity is something more than giving money. Charity is also about giving when you have nothing to give. Mother Theresa said it was easy to give some coins when you had many, what was harder was to give your last coin. I really took this on board. I realized this statement was a truth and when you hear the truth it flows into every cell of your body and sits there being configured. Of course, she was not only talking about money but about your time. Giving time when you say you have none forces you to look at the content of your day. Einstein was disappointed to find that time was indeed relative. He had hoped to 'discover' time. Your day may drag slowly, while your friend next door can't find enough hours in the day. The time on the clock is the same for you both, and it ticks away the same. Placing your mind in the moment slows it down. Falling in love does this, as does an accident. People say, "It felt like everything was in slow motion." When this happens, you can see each frame of time and its content. Mindlessness either allows you to be bored or you are asleep and time is squandered. I have an insane timetable, a very demanding job and, as a single mother, four children to provide for, but I always have time for mentoring, volunteering and my friends. When I sit, I sit, when I'm with them, I am with them.

———— • • • ————

Time is measured by its content.
Make time for others.
Give your time, not just your money.

———— • • • ————

12 Take a Look at Your Reflection and Consider the Lines You See Etched There by Your Life so Far

"A face tells a million stories," my Mother would say. I used to think about this when I was little and wondered if she meant that the face could speak because it had a mouth. She explained that smiling a lot caused the lines on a face and she showed me her lines around her eyes and mouth. She then pointed out the lines on her forehead where she worried about things and I began to look at my own face in the same way. "So if I smile," I said, "these lines show the world that I'm someone who is pretty happy, and these lines up here will be the ones that tell me, and the world, that I'm worried or scared. Can I hide these lines, Mummy?"

"Yes of course you can," Mom replied. "But if you do, then people won't be able to read your face and all its stories."

As a middle-aged woman I think that cosmetic surgery and Botox just let your face lie and make up stories. The Australian Aborigines believe all white people lie, that they wear a mask and don't know how to tell the truth. I think about this a lot, especially when dealing with certain situations where the truth, the whole truth, can be the hardest way to go.

13 Place Your Hand on Your Heart and Say, "I Breathe, Therefore I Am"

I love what I do. It allows me to meet people from all walks of life. But even my own inspiring work *is* work in the end and can consume every day. I had a big health warning in 2010 and I ended up in hospital having a brain scan after doctors thought I might have had a stroke. This was a big shock to me and a bigger shock to those who live and work with me. I had recently lost my darling Mother to a particularly evil cancer of the gall bladder and had kept myself sane by working, to help me stay focused. I nursed Mom at home until I couldn't carry her. I knew every part of her body in the months I had her with me. I washed her, clothed and medicated her. I watched her fight the idea of death and saw her fear and anger. She was the most amazing person: full of smiles and passion for her acting, and her endeavor to live forever was a mission! My brother said that he thought she would live to 110 and then die in her sleep after a brilliant performance. We all thought that, and Mom, more than any of us, truly believed that she deserved that. Her life as a child was wonderful and she used to say, rather shamefully, that some of her happiest years were during the Second World War! She lived it from the age of 11 to 17: very formative years, she would say! She died a horrible and undignified death: so unfair.

My Mother was at home with me, dying, and I needed to make a new DVD. I took a night out and asked the film crew to set up two cameras and go away. I so needed to do my own Yoga, to step out of the role of carer and reach a place with no pain. I did a two hour self-practice, stood up afterwards, called in the crew and left.

Mum never saw that film but it's interesting how it's one of my most popular DVDs. People always say there is a special 'feel' about it.

I managed to work 24/7 on my school and travelled before and after her death in a professional capacity. Keeping busy with what I loved doing saved me from falling apart and being useless. My Mother had always supported my work ethic because she knew this was who I was.

Her acting was her greatest personal achievement, together with being the Mayor of Southwark. She understood that motherhood was a joy to us both, but that we were just individuals before we had children and that in order to remain happy, one needs to find that person again.

It occurred to me, one day after she had died, that I had become not myself but an extension of myself. I had become my job and I had lost some thread of my own reality.

• • •

I actually said to a friend, "I work therefore I am!"

• • •

It was clear to me then that I had lost my way. Work, in my case, is a very real part of me but it is only part of me; it is not

'I'. I stopped teaching so many classes and backed off. I knew it was a time to heal and that if I didn't give myself that time I might very well be on my way to a head-on collision with the Universe!

So I placed my hand on my heart and said

●———————— ● ● ● ————————●

"I breathe, therefore I am."

●———————— ● ● ● ————————●

14 Sit Down and Don't Do Anything

OK, so this is the easy part. Hilarious! I think that this is the most difficult aspect of my life. I had a really horrible evening with my youngest daughter. I remember clearly being 16 and I can remember how I felt, too. I hated being talked to by my parents. It was a physical revulsion. I didn't want them to know anything about my life. Nothing! The rage I felt was a glowing red, like the embers of a fire. I was about to blow up all the time, an inner explosion of frustration and anger at the people who said they loved me yet seemed to be the only ones who didn't understand me. The thing is, I can also still remember how I felt when I told them these feelings: how I screamed, and one time swore at my Mother. I remember it because it felt awful and shameful. My Father's strict Arab upbringing meant he wanted to give me a good hiding when I behaved like this but I learned to run as I continued to abuse him! My Mother, on the other hand, was a well-balanced, stoical person, with great integrity. She would just tell me, after I calmed down, that no matter what, she loved me. That would bring a bittersweet feeling of shame and exhaustion, as well as relief. I honestly thought I was the same sort of mother. But my daughter is not me, though she is, in many ways, exactly like me. She is influenced by all sorts of things I had no idea existed. Sitting down and saying nothing, as a parent, seems impossible, but sometimes I just have to sit still and not become a part of the drama.

15 Stay Still and Empty Your Mind

It is at times like this that it is useful to stop still, as long as it's safe to do so, and breathe very slowly! If you feel overheated, imagine your head depositing its contents into a bin. Imagine you're an hourglass timer if you feel harried, and let the petals of whatever flower resonates with you rest in your belly if you're feeling fragile, all this to the silent accompaniment of the breath.

16

Open up your face
Lift the shadows
Rub the dust from your lids
Sparkle, Shine, Light up!
You are the first thing you see reflected back to you

17 My Mind is an Empty Space and my Body the Rainbow

Feel the Earth pulse under your bottom
It's been there the whole time
If you have a heart, so does the Earth

Suffocate it and it struggles to breathe
You and the Earth are one, or the very thing you rely on will
  leave you without support
Sit like a young child, not like an old dog
No matter if you are 100 years old
Stretch the spine upwards and think of the tree you planted
  once
The Earth and water nourished the tree and it grew strong
  and straight
Lay on your plate the colors of the rainbow for your physical
  body
Eat the rainbow and realize the colors feed your subtle
  other body
Don't let your mind dismiss this knowledge
It's trying hard to make you say, "No, this is no-sense"
So the real work begins on the busy mind and its hold on you

Let's start at the physical level. We are all made of rainbows, whether it be reflections of the sky's rainbow in our eyes or the feeling of a rainbow in the heart when someone begins to fall in love with us and we with them. It's a connection, a bridge.

That rainbow brings us back to our childhood, to our past memories and our first encounter with love. This often manifests as the mother. If there is no mother figure in our life, then we are forced to reach much deeper into our own pool of resources, long before we're ready to do so. Allow your life, for a few days, weeks, years or a lifetime, to reflect the idea of the rainbow. The seven colors of the Chakras are the same as our rainbow. All these colors merged become white, become light and feed us from the inside out, as opposed to physical food that feeds from the outside in. The simplest advice I gave my children was to fill their plates with color, and then they could be sure to be eating well. This worked as much when they were tiny as when they went off to University!

18 Are We Strangers or are We Human?

My Mother was forever reminding me that each and every one of us has a 'story'. In other words, few of us escape pain, heartache and fear along life's way.

I remember, as a child, thinking a lot about other people's stories and wondering what they were. I liked to talk to strangers and I learned to ask good questions. Insightful questions are like a magnifying glass, revealing people's private inner worlds.

Trust comes into its own realm when people allow you a glimpse behind the scenes. "It's an honor and a privilege," my Father would say. He was a deeply private person and held his pain like an injured child.

I used to think, what happens to us when we hold onto pain? I believe I know now. Looking at your own dark space, don't dismiss it as a weak place. This dark space, where no one talks or touches or hears, is our own private hell. It can take a lifetime, in fact, many lifetimes, before we find the courage to look into the dark mirror, the strength necessary to hold it in front of us and allow our vision to steady.

Never looking at ourselves can hold us back from moving forward. Terrifying things may cause an emotional paralysis. We are rooted but unable to breathe, embedded but unable to grow. Stuck. Jammed. Held down. Squeezed to death.

This is why we often don't look at ourselves, our 'self'. So begin again to

Open your eyes wide and just see without looking
Just hear without listening
Place a hand to your heart and feel without searching
Reach out without touching; just sense the moment
Sense the moment, experience the place and wake up

19 Delusion or Illusion?

Being Alice in Wonderland or Aladdin Sane is an imaginary idea. Is it? Sanity, image, poetic license, all of these concepts are ways of telling the truth by creating a drama. Stepping out of our scene demands that we accept we are taking part in it in the first place. Accepting that we are indeed playing a role leads us to explore the part and why we chose it. Sometimes we are gifted with a flash of insight, which enables us to recognize our devastating scenario as one of God's jokes. We manage, just for a split second, to stand apart and laugh at our misfortune, and allow others to laugh and share in the joke! Taking things personally places us right back in our drama and one way to avoid that pitfall is by consciously choosing a role. Another is to decide not to take part at all or to be in the audience or to simply be the stagehand standing in the wings, observing the play but not taking part.

I always say to my children and students, "Just jump in, join the group and commit to whatever you do. Otherwise it's like going to a party and not taking your coat off. You stand and watch but don't feel the pulse of that particular scene. Asking you to be fully involved is not the same as you getting embroiled in an episode of *Coronation Street*, this is real life!

20 Take a Part

I was six months pregnant with my first son and allowing myself time to grow and nurture us both. I saw a Tai Chi course running in London and thought that it might be a fun and interesting body discipline for me during this time. The Tai Chi Master was a very well-known Chinese Californian, with the directness only Americans have. He began the day by telling us a story.

There was a daisy, tightly closed, still a bud, but its potential was to be beautiful. As spring came the bud began to open and each petal in turn presented itself. However, one or two petals decided they wouldn't do the same as the others; refusing their natural duty, they stayed curled up. The daisy's potential of being beautiful was ruined, because it needed all the petals to reach its full potential.

I know for a fact that story was meant for me. It was the first time I realized I may be arrogant! If I stood on the outside looking in I was not performing my duty as a group member. I lost out; we all lost out. Take part wholeheartedly not half-heartedly, commit!

• • •

Learn to put pride in its right place and admit you are scared.
Do not block personal growth.

• • •

21 Self-motivation and the Big 'E' – Effort

I was talking to my nephew today, about those who take but never give. I was giving him a lecture on getting on with his coursework for his chance to get to university. He has had a lot of bad luck but he has also made wrong decisions. I was listening to a song from the 50s and 60s, a doo-wop song called *I'm not a juvenile delinquent*. It's about doing the right thing, and being happy, because being good is easy and being bad is hard. I thought that if we told all young people this from early on, they would believe it as much as they believe 'being good is hard'.

I was telling my nephew that he had spent a lot of his youth taking from others, and that he had naively thought this would help him accumulate what he wanted. I pointed out to him that those who take get nothing back; in fact they lose all they take. On the other hand, givers get back a lot of energy and money: actions are like boomerangs. Takers lose the boomerang; it always gets away, while those who give keep getting that boomerang back.

22 Money Matters

Take money, for instance. It's energy, just like anything else. If we despise it, we often have little of it. If we earn it honestly, it can grow, but if we hold onto it and become greedy, it can kill us. Money is like blood: it has to flow to remain healthy. If blood gets congealed or stuck in an area of the body, we get ill.

23 Reach Your Potential

I ask all my children and my nieces and nephews to consider their own potential. If it's so easy to think badly of our own talents and achievements, then why can't we turn it around and believe in ourselves?

It's like believing in God. We don't have to see the Divine to believe it exists; yet people have to see results to believe they are achievable. This has always puzzled me from a very young age.

Are we deluded or living an illusion? We do know what the right action is but for some reason we just don't have that extra push we need to achieve our dreams.

A dream will only ever be a dream until we make it a reality
After that you have no dreams because you are part of them

24 I Honestly Believe There is No Such Thing as Impossible

I know everything is possible because I do it every day. Each day I make something happen that seems to others to be too difficult. I would like to thank my parents and everyone involved in my creation for allowing me the courage to believe in the possibility of moving mountains.

———— • • • ————

Be champions for others who cannot champion themselves. Be the one to say, "Take my hand, I will walk with you."

———— • • • ————

25

Say nothing if your words are not tinted with Love
Make no moves if those moves are not from the heart
Touch no one if that touch is not as light as the air
Carry yourself with humility and without fear
Walk through life with grace and power but never with arrogance
Sing from your soul, let your voice lift the heavens and all that are in them
Life is a gift; it is our duty to enjoy it

26 When to Help, and When to Hold Back

The problem with that 'helping hand' is that sometimes it's hard to imagine ever being able to let go. It's interesting, for example, how children in the same family, though they all had the same love, upbringing and chances, turn out so differently. That's probably the most difficult aspect of parenting, knowing that they will never be yours, either in temperament, vision, talent or skill. Often they are better, in fact, but make choices you would not have made. When do we walk away and when can we stay?

It's just as interesting to watch adults and their parenting from the point of view of a child. My parents fought all the time, well, a lot of the time, and it was mostly after we had gone to bed. The bedroom light was out but the light on the landing created a luminous line under the door. This made the dark even darker. Noises, voices, furniture, silence. Sounds were muffled to save us from hearing. It made it worse. All the spaces between those sounds led to my naive imagination filling those gaps. Those imaginings carried powerful emotions, leading me to move to a conscious decision. I remember thinking that I would never let that happen to me! No arguments, no threats, no feeling of woman being lower than man. A rage started to burn inside of me, and I keep to my word most of the time. D.I.V.O.R.C.E. I did do well though, I am 'Happily Divorced' and we remain good friends. Result!

"We stayed together for the children." My goodness, what a sentence to lay at a child's door. Well I wish you hadn't and especially not for me. Why didn't you ask me what I wanted? P.E.A.C.E. But I also saw my parents get through in the end. It's something, as modern men and women, which we find hard to understand. I honestly don't know what is right. I've done what I needed to do at the time and I always felt I was saving myself from the drudgery of being a woman. I did the 'Holy Mother' and loved it, but I'm also the 'Holy Father', the carer, and the hunter-gatherer.

27 Unto One's Self be True

Each step we take in this world leaves a mark on it, which cannot be helped. We need to forgive, not just others but ourselves. This is exactly the conversation Krishna had with Arjuna in the Baghavad Gita. We cannot help leaving some debris in our wake when traveling a path we were destined to walk. This 'soul debris' is called duty, *Dharma*, no choice, the only choice, and the best we can do; it has many names. Be honest and take courage—it's the only option when dealing with the family and all those separate minds.

28 The Long and Winding Road

I have had the highest highs and the lowest lows. I've had the courage to drop off the edge of sanity just long enough for me to touch my toes into another world. I know I live my life on the edge of that cliff, with my toes finely balanced, while my body adopts the pose of an athletic ballerina or that of a graceful footballer. I stay still, one toe on the edge, arms lifted and my leg extended. I can see far below me and I see nothing at all but clouds of memory. I do not look behind because I know where I have been. I look straight ahead at the horizon; it's always the darkest just before the dawn.

29 When Falling, Dive

Once I fell, and I wanted to fall. I said, "To hell with this I've had enough." As I fell, everything was very slow, like moving through honey. I was Alice in Wonderland, falling down the rabbit hole. I could see bits of my everyday life as I fell, pots and pans, cups and saucers, gardens and gates, windows and my reflection. I could have stopped if I had wanted to. As I fell I knew I had a choice, a choice to fall on my feet, the choice to fall on my head. Right then I wanted to experience terrible physical pain that matched the emotional pain of DEPRESSION.

30 Stand up

All my life I thought everyone was depressed: that depression was a 'dark place' where all of us, at some time, curled up and were motionless, blind and mute: that this was a world inside the head that cut us off from our physical body...our very own DARK PLACE.

What I discovered one day, while talking to my sister, is that we don't all have a dark place we visit, and that it seems we don't all suffer from depression. She had had terrible things happen to her, but she wasn't depressed. That was a huge eyes-opening-wide moment. My brain cranked its cogs and it started to move. REALISATION!

I got up after I put the phone down. I stood in the middle of the room. I was alone. I raised my hand and I said, out loud to the wall, "My name is Anne-Marie and I suffer from depression." That was the beginning of my journey in and out of my dark place. It took hard work and commitment to realize I could control the feelings that rose up like a fire, like panic, no...terror. I began to realize that these feelings were different from the depression. The depression made me feel bad about myself. I would be in so deep I couldn't remember one single person who loved me or cared about me. Actually, this is unique to depression. If you are simply down, you can remember, but when you're depressed, you honestly have no memory of anything but the place, space, moment you're in now. It took me years to separate anxiety from depression, then depression from panic.

Panic attacks can be so random, a tsunami, an earthquake, an overwhelming emotional experience, and they should never be ignored, made light of or explained away. I now know that these are a symptom of deeper underlying factors. A personal journey will involve unpacking years of feelings that are jumbled up together. I see this as putting all the wrong colors together in one wash and ending up with grey. Taking each part of the trauma apart is a deconstruction of events, each part a clue to a puzzle.

I honestly believe that if we are given the time and the support we can start to heal our lives.

31 Being Here Now

This has been misrepresented as a good place to be. But being here now means being in that moment of terror, too. Yes, of course, ideally, being here now would be ecstatic and the place that feels liberating. Is it then a HAPPY PLACE? No, it's also a fact that we need to be in the moment, accepting the feeling of the space we're in. This could be the depression, the loneliness, the isolation, the voice inside that tells you, 'you're no good', 'you're not deserving of love', and 'you're not cherished'. Conclusion: A skill must be found to help get through this passage without PAINKILLERS.

32 This Too Shall Pass

The following is a good illustration of how to help yourself or someone else 'get through' this dark passage and move toward the light. The Maharaja suffered from dark spells that caused him to feel desperate and lonely and unworthy of his status. In a word, he suffered from depression. He called upon all his wisest men to go and find a remedy and he threatened to cut off their heads if they returned without it. Most never returned for fear of losing their heads! His oldest Vizier took it upon himself to find a cure for his master's dark spells. He rode around the country, listening to folk and seeking out demons and magicians and apothecaries, but with no luck. On his way back home, weary and full of dread, he came upon a clearing in the wood. Here was an old man and a young boy and it seemed as though the boy was apprenticed to the old man. The boy was sobbing hard but the old man was unmoved.

"Boy," he said, "stop crying, stop your wailing, be still, as this, too, shall pass."

Hearing those words, the Vizier rode hard, back to his master.

"Well," the Maharaja demanded, "give me the remedy, the potion, the herbs to cast off this dark spell."

The Vizier knelt down, bowing his head, he said, "Oh Master, this too shall pass, as any other day."

"Ah," said the Maharaja. And he saw that indeed he felt the clouds lift and the sun begin to warm his face. All things are transient and it's a choice to suffer.

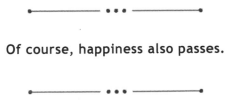

Of course, happiness also passes.

Conclusion: Moderation must prevail in all things, including suffering and happiness. Stop sticking labels onto your feelings. I have done this myself: that's why no one cares, I am unlovable, I am invisible, I am a bad person. In this way we begin to create and weave a web around us; it's just an illusion.

33

And it seemed to me as I raised my face
That the chasm of the sky opened and both thunder and
rain fell
It fell hard and I was cleansed
I was of Hope
And ready to begin again

34 Thoughts Create Emotions

Thinking about a lover and the last time you made love brings those feelings on, a shiver down the back as the energy flows from the base of the spine. The thought, smell, or photo of a mother or father who has died, or a child, brings with it that very raw and real emotion of pain; the heart aches with it. Yet a few moments ago, you were feeling fine. Again, it is a choice, but it's tough to accept that, because a part of us needs the pain to remind us of our own fragile life.

35 Take the Happiness and Say Thank You

Why is it so difficult to accept happiness, I wonder? It's so good to see people who are comfortable in their own body. As a ballet dancer I had to starve every day and I began to equate my image with my happiness. If I put on a couple of pounds I hated myself and wanted to die. The only time I was able to enjoy putting on weight was when I was pregnant. I loved seeing my body grow. It was one of the first times I ever considered I was worth something because the focus was on another life, not mine. I'm much better now but will always be scarred by the suffering a dancer is placed under and accepts as a part of the job. However, at least I'm aware of the ghost of that time in my mind; I can see it on the horizon and change direction.

36 Signposts and How to Read Them

Life offers us many opportunities for change. Often we are blind to the signs on the road, sometimes we choose to ignore the warning lights and decide to suffer or fail. I was explaining this to my younger daughter, who often says something negative when I say something positive to her. "You're allowing that mind voice to put you down and destroy your own potential. Why?" She answered that she knew what she was doing, and that part of that was how she felt about herself.

"I may never be anything," she said, "so this way I can't fail!"

As a mother, this is devastating to hear but it's my duty to help her now, not run away. "Please remember every day that you are loved, deeply loved," I offered. As a parent, you know that you're clutching at anything to make yourself feel better. I can only guide and shine a light in the right direction, no more. The key is knowing when to stop giving advice and to leave the child to find their own way.

37 Learning to Fail

There is a big movement in Sweden at this time, focused on celebrating failure. Talking to young people, this has resonated with them.

It takes some pressure away from only achieving success and illustrates that all those who do succeed have experienced a lot of failure, disappointment and doubt.

It's OK to be enough and it's downright essential to fail, to battle and strive. This builds muscle for the work ahead and the understanding that, like all things in life, if we accept our failures we may be able to see our successes.

38 Life is a Cappuccino

Some like it with a dusting of chocolate, some without. Either way it is a ritual that attaches the action to satisfaction. It must be my Arab-Anglo heritage that attaches to coffee and tea rituals as a ceremony of togetherness or aloneness.

39 Embracing Love Includes Loving Ourselves

Samantha in 'Sex in the City', when leaving Smith (her lover, for those uneducated amongst us) said, "Smith, I love you, but I love me more." Classic! I actually said that myself to a class of students I had taught for ten years in response to their cry of, "Anne-Marie you can't give up the class, we need it!" I replied, "I love you all, but I love me more!" Yeah!!! I was so proud of myself!

But, I have wandered off the subject.

Let's return to how to deal with the low times in a practical way. Sit with a straight spine; sit still and in a comfortable place. Place the back of the hands on the knees. Close the eyes and watch the breath. Breathe in very slowly and breathe out even slower. Let the thoughts settle. Think of an egg timer and the sand at the top as all the thoughts in the mind. As the breath gets regular and slows, the thoughts drop, like sand, to the lower body, the belly, and become the breath. Now you are holding your breath in the bowl of the belly. Breathe in and out. Now notice where your depression and loneliness are. The pain

43

may be in your heart, chest or belly. Maybe it's in your arms or legs. Maybe it's in your mind? Don't think, just notice.

40 Do Nothing

This is the opposite of what we often do when we are low.

We usually do one of these:

- Talk to a friend, going round and round the garden
- Drink a bottle of wine to drown our sorrows
- Have a lot of sex with lovers, friends or strangers, never having a satisfying orgasm
- Smoke a lot till we hate ourselves and we smell of that hate
- Binge on chocolate and crisps to hate ourselves more than we hate others

But stop! None of these are the cure; they are delaying tactics, because facing our real pain and why we feel like this is terrifying.

In a moment of emotional crisis, try doing nothing
Just wait, and eventually those scary fears pass because you
*   gave them no attention*
Fear feeds itself on fear, not acceptance

41

Thoughts simply create emotions
When a crisis slaps you down or weakens you, go through
*   the motions*

Get up, get dressed, clean your teeth, eat
As you focus on these daily routines
Your heart will begin to settle down and your strength will
  recover

42 Honor the Brave

Listening to the radio one day in 2013, I heard that a female war correspondent was killed in Syria. No one outside the world of journalism was aware that this woman reported atrocities and horrors because she believed we should know the truth. She was only a year older than myself. Her face adorned the front page of the Times. She had been a Sunday Times reporter. I heard someone say, "I didn't even know she existed or that she did the work she did till now, now that she is dead." Amen.

43 Courage

Both my parents were human rights activists, and again, no one knew what they had to endure to make people sit up and listen. They also made sure we knew what was going on in the world. There is a magazine written by women who have been imprisoned for their resistance to the despotic regimes they live under. One story will never leave me and it was not unusual, in fact, had my Mother not smuggled us out of Iraq back in 1960, then it would have happened to her. Let's call the woman Samira. Samira's husband was a political activist. He resisted the crushing regime's attempts to silence the people by means of abuse, torture and imprisonment. One night the soldiers raided Samira's house and took her husband and her children. She was left in utter torment for 24 hours. On their return, the soldiers took her. She was put in a cell, alone, next to the one with her children. The youngest was still breast-feeding. They starved the children, forcing her to endure their weeping and moaning, and then, the final, terrible silence. This was an attempt to make Samira incriminate her husband and the people he worked with. Many women like Samira let their children die for the common good, in other words, to save the children and men of many more women. What would you have done? I often flinched from reading these stories. My Mother said, "If these women can suffer and tell their story, the least you can do is to respect them enough to read it." Again, Amen.

I am no more
My body is flesh and my mind a forest of moving images
Touch my body and it burns with fear
Pierce my mind and it shrieks with terror
Clothe my soul with a mantle of peace and kiss my lips
*   though they sing no more*

44 Sticks and Stones Leave Marks and Words Leave Scars

I have memories from a very young age, maybe because I feel as though I have had two distinctly separate lives. The first was only up to the age of six, in 1950s Iraq. When I was born, the country was flourishing culturally and educationally, yet it was still in the dark ages for those in poverty. Both my paternal grandparents could neither read nor write. Somehow, they had the vision to support my Father's endeavors to study in England. To this day I have no idea how they did it. I never asked him! So much is lost when our parents die. When I think about those early years, it is all hot colors, strong smells, food, and mostly being outside. When I consider my first memories of England, they are all of soft greys, some reds, noisy traffic and always being inside. I had to stop speaking Iraqi to help me integrate more easily and had to adapt to things like wearing shoes all day. The smell of chamomile I now only smelled in tea. Yet the valleys around Southern Iraq are covered with the tiny, white and yellow chamomile. I was small, so the flowers came up to my thighs. I used to wander off alone, very happy to meet no one. I would come across some mud huts and see mothers feeding their babies and women making flat bread in the large clay ovens. I only knew I was a girl when my brother was born. That was when I was forced to take another look at my then happy life. Boys came first; girls came second, and that was that. My paternal Grandfather doted on me and I adored him. He would wander off with the other men to the chai shop to sit, talk, smoke and generally do what men like to do best, be with other men. After my brother was born, I felt things I had never felt before: jealously, rage, indignation and rejection. I must have been three and a half, and I saw my Poppa walk off to the chai shop with my eighteen-month-old brother, I ran after him thinking he had forgotten me. Instead he said, "How could you shame me? Girls are not allowed at the chai shop. Go back now. Shame, shame!" I turned around. I was so hurt I stopped dead still, paralyzed with shock and confusion. I can still remember it all and feel it.

My brother, who has served a long and hard prison sentence, reminded me that

— • • • —

People rarely remember what you say, but always remember how you made them feel.

— • • • —

45 Who Am I?

How do we become uniquely us? How much of our past really belongs to us? How many memories are uniquely our own? Each one of us has heard stories, either from our mother's knee or from some other source that embedded ideas into our consciousness. Patterns of behavior can start to create deep grooves, even though we personally have never experienced anything that might instigate that particular behavior. In Vedic philosophy, those habits or grooves are called *Samsaras*. This is easy to remember because of the scar that the name *Samsara* alludes to.

I had a friend who was a conservative American, I suppose. She was classic in style, in both her clothes and her home. She played the cello and was silent and deep. It took a long time to get to know her.

She told me one day that she had decided to see a therapist to help her with unacceptable, and also unfamiliar, behavior. It transpired that her parents had been alcoholics and the behavior she was manifesting was theirs, so she was behaving like an alcoholic although she wasn't one in reality. As a child she had simply 'copied' their behavior, much as a child would copy a parent's smoking habit, without understanding it or connecting to it. I found that fascinating. So her *Samsaras* were imprinted rather than experienced.

It felt very important to me to try to understand this better and I spent time researching.

Adult children of alcoholics have a fear of people who are in authority, people who are angry, and do not take personal criticism very well. Often they misinterpret assertiveness for anger. Therefore, they are constantly seeking approval of others whilst losing their identities in the process. Frequently they isolate themselves. Often, these adult children will acquire the characteristics of alcoholics, even if they never drink themselves. They can be in denial, develop poor coping strategies, have an inability to problem solve and form dysfunctional relationships.

They will do anything to save a relationship rather than face the pain of abandonment, even if the relationship is unhealthy.

As I read these statements, it seemed like a huge responsibility, having children. We can so easily burden them with our own demons. We both had young ones and suddenly I felt really fortunate to have sorted out some of my demons before I had children...ha! I say that...but no sooner do you have a thought like that and bam! God delivers one of his jokes. I returned home, pondering my friend's past and present. I walked in, saw the mess in the kitchen, my husband reading the paper, and flipped! "So you think you are done?" the Divine seems to say, before delivering one humungous challenge and pulling the rug out from under your feet. "Try this for size!"

46

Dear Divine,
I positively and carefully
Place my mind at your feet
I am noticing each step
Conscious of the Earth
Am slow in mind and action
...on a day like today when Man, Woman and Child could
*   make a difference*
In Me are the Holy Child, the Mother and the Father
Amen

47 A Path is a Personal Journey

I was walking around Waterlow Park in North London back in 1985 with my first son, then only a few months old. I loved that park: it was heavenly, on top of a hill, next to Highgate Cemetery and just by a really commanding Catholic church. I bumped into a very sweet Hindu elder walking around the pond there. I don't know how we started talking but he was telling me how he had had Jehovah's Witnesses at the door. He had told them quietly and respectfully that his faith was Hindu. One of the Witnesses had tried to put a foot in the door, causing the gentleman to feel afraid. He said, "Why can't they respect that I have found my way?" I really resonated with this observation.

● — ● ● ● — ●

Respect is tantamount to acceptance, tolerance and compassion.

● — ● ● ● — ●

48 Within You and Without You

I was watching a program about the late George Harrison, of The Beatles. They were talking about the album *Sgt. Pepper's Lonely Hearts Club Band*. The Beatles were saying how it gave them the chance to be another band and gave them permission to sound different and to create a new personality. After listening to the lyrics, something I never did because I was a drummer and only heard the riffs, I realized George had really understood and aligned with Yoga and Hindu philosophy and that the effects of meditation had resonated deeply within him. He wrote a song called *'Within You Without You.'* It explained simply and beautifully how God (the Divine) is here, there and everywhere. As a practicing Yoga devotee I understood his language.

The late TV presenter David Frost was interviewing the band and he really was both sympathetic and interested. He did an excellent job of helping the audience glimpse something of the philosophy behind meditation, while at the same time asking questions that delved a lot deeper. You can talk to many musicians from the rock scene back in the 60s, 70s and 80s and find very similar examples of life-changing experiences while practicing meditation.

49 Silence is Something You Invite into Your Space

A noisy day can be made silent by standing still inside a thought that has been left suspended. Breathing slowly and deeply while your thought now drifts to settle in the belly. You become still, and with that stillness you invite silence into your space.

50 Asking for Silence

Prayer and contemplation are not the same as the 'Silence that surpasses all understanding' because to think a word of prayer or to contemplate the words of a saint or scholar needs mental effort: movement of thought. Watching is a path to silence. Stop playing the role and lay the script of life down. Simply 'be' in your space and let silence enter. One of my favorite people is Sister Wendy, a devout Catholic nun, who mostly lives in seclusion. She goes out into the world only in response to invitations to speak or expound on art, which she expresses through her spiritual meditations and deep contemplations. It was through her writings that I began to understand the idea of asking silence to enter my life. I realized it wasn't a case of 'finding silence' but inviting it to enter you. This made so much sense; it really was like a light being turned on.

•————— • • • —————•

Guru (teacher): One who takes you from darkness to light.

•————— • • • —————•

51

Meditation is not an art or a skill
It is a falling into a tiny gap in the conscious mind
A slipping into a shaft of that consciousness
That is not a place of knowing but a place of not knowing
I was blind and now I see I am blind

52 Learn That There is More Than One Way to Travel the Mind

When travelling around India back in 1984, I came to a tiny place in Rajasthan. I met with a female Swami who taught me to meditate with my eyes open. I found this very difficult. I honestly thought it could not be right to meditate this way. She sat next to me and just looked, no movement of eye but just looking. She explained that the noise and movement in India was one of the reasons to mediate; it was survival after all! So one could meditate within the bazaar of color, smell and sound and be in a place by really feeling wide awake, taking in all the landscape as a whole, not just a part. It can be described as a stage, I think. When the performance ends, the curtain closes but there is still a lot going on behind it, even though you have switched off the lights, sounds and action. Shakespeare understood this; life is a stage and we the performers. There are roles we may choose to play; a drama we can accept or not; a part in a mystical version of *Eastenders*.

53 Living Life with Ultimate Joy

Sister Wendy Beckett (British hermit, consecrated virgin and art historian) has a favorite book by Dorothy Day, an American Catholic, who began the magazine called *The Catholic Worker*. She worked endlessly for her community. The title of the book is *The Duty of Delight*. Sister Wendy commented that, "It is our duty to enjoy life. It's a gift." Religion can so often suffocate this joy of life, which is, after all, God-Given. The idea of suffering is certainly the Western way. The Dalai Lama writes, "There is only one way, the way of happiness." East and West, Ying and Yang, Night and Day, Shiva and Shakti; all of these opposites are paths for the mind; they must meet somewhere. The human psyche finds it so easy to see the negative. Our work needs to begin in seeing the good things in life, and time to reflect is a privilege in itself.

•————— • • • —————•

Somewhere there is a place for us.

•————— • • • —————•

54 Walking on the Line

"East of Easy,
South of Simple,
West of where I wanna be.
We all know the North is way too cold.
Meet me in the middle
...
We can have a little paradise of our very own."

I heard this song, *East of Easy*, by 'The Red Bullets' today. When I heard the chorus I thought, the path to the middle must be the hardest road. Why? Because there is no map that shows the 'Middle'.

55 Listening for Messages

I had a long discourse today with my younger brother, who has suffered a deep-rooted mental illness for some time. He is in his miraculous metamorphic state now, having seen the delusions as just that and no more. He has always been spiritually interested in both Eastern and Western religion and we were talking about God.

He had once been a Hare Krishna and came back to his Christian roots through his illness (or times of 3rd dimension, as I often call it). Our background is Syrian Orthodox and I call him a Hare 'Kristian!' We each embraced new belief systems around the same time. I was finding Yoga as he was rediscovering his Christian roots. He got into drug use to cope with overwhelming issues that he now cannot remember and I came out of my sex, drugs and rock'n'roll lifestyle and into Yoga.

We softly argued about what God was. He said God is in human form, therefore we look like God. I thought God was all pervading and was therefore not an image but a spark that splintered into each of us and that was the 'Light' or the 'Holy Spirit'. What was so interesting was that our own beliefs had stemmed from parents who were atheists, politically active and yet the most spiritual people I knew. We ended our lovely, sunny discourse on a ritual for bringing people together and agreed we would have to reconcile our differences over a second cappuccino!

56 Know your Name

My maiden name is KHACHIK. As an Armenian and a Syrian Orthodox Christian its interpretation has no dualities. Khachik means 'crucifix'. I didn't learn this for many years. One day I asked my Father about the meaning of his name, Abdulahad. He told me it was 'Slave of God'. It was then he explained the significance of our surname. For me, the crucifix is a shield. I can remember thinking I had a lot to live up to and my name would always keep me safe.

57 Faith for the Brave

What do people who don't have a faith do? Do they explore science? It has always been interesting to me that I was brought up in duality, my Christian Orthodox roots and politics. My parents were communists and I never once felt that they put me in any danger living what they believed in. Once upon a time, here in England, having a faith put you in danger. If you were Catholic, you had to hide that fact or risk death. This persecution made people hold tighter to their faith and to their political views, made them stronger not weaker. There needs to be a quiet resolve to walk the walk of death and to speak the unspoken. Courage? Yes, but also an unprecedented belief for these courageous people that they were on the path they were meant to be on. We are all amazed and in awe of those brave souls who knew that there was no going back. I was always fascinated by the life of Joan of Arc. My Mother had the same name and my favorite Aunt in Lebanon was called Jean D'Arc. Joan of Arc was 19 when she died and I have often imagined myself in her place. How brave would I be? How alone must she have been? And yet her conviction was so powerful.

A silent sublime radiance arose in her eyes as she walked
towards the end of her day
A simple child clothed in humility and maybe ignorance?
Where is my Mother? Where is my Father?
The same words and feelings Jesus asked himself as he died
on the cross
Am I alone, am I abandoned?
And Yet I raise my eyes to the heavens and understand
everything
All is as it should be

58 I Don't Know What I Am

I asked my children to do their best to reach their potential.

My son asked me, "How do I do that?"

"Put one foot in front of the other," I told him, "don't look back unless you know it's for the purpose of learning from what has gone. If there is a hole in the ground then ignore it and step over. Reaching your potential is about believing you have a purpose in life and never giving up until you know you have found it."

Trust that you are already on route to your purpose. Sometimes looking for it is when you lose your way. My Mother had this wonderful rhyme.

"Follow love and it will flee; flee love and it will follow thee."
-*English proverb*

In other words, stop asking and just believe.

59 Same Subject Different Translation!

My younger brother and I were discussing religion again (our favorite subject) and God and the universe, over our weekly Wednesday morning coffee date. He is a Christian and I'm an 'all that makes sense and sits with me' person. He was discussing The Son of God and I was discussing The Sun of God. He asked me if I didn't accept that in the beginning there was light. Actually, I do believe this and it's scientifically acceptable, as is the Divine. Acceptance is the big word in any faith and I honestly believe that science and spiritual teachings can be brothers. A teacher, a leader, a scholar or a child – in their present moment – gives us light.

The Sun of God is such an interesting truth. If we go back to the time when we had no idea that beyond the horizon, over the mountain, or across the sea were others living simple lives, though there were great thinkers, they still only had their own environment to tell them of things greater than themselves. If I had lived in the mountains of Afghanistan in ages past, I would have prayed for a harvest of apricots. If the yield turned out to be poor, then I might have considered I had done something to anger the sun or the rain. If I had lived in Bangladesh when there were floods that swept homes and people away, I might have believed that the gods were punishing me.

If I lived in the mountains, in the snow, and my business

depended on the snow, then if it did not arrive, again, I might consider I was being punished. Religion, faith and trust are all natural, and just as real, no matter where we live. But for some, the idea that we could ever have come to believe God had a Son in human form is quite appalling. The Koran speaks of this, as does the Torah. These two faiths do not believe Jesus to be the Son of God. But I am sure he is THE SUN OF GOD.

— • • —

We need a constant in our lives.
The sun rising and the sun setting is that safe constant.
Could the apocalypse be that the sun did not rise
and therefore we remain in Darkness?
As we know, Darkness is Ignorance.

— • • —

60 Same Intention Different Language

When I was a child, I was woken every single morning with the sound of "Allah Akbar," the call to prayers of the Muslim faith. I love that sound and that call. As a baby, growing up in Iraq, I felt very safe. The reason? The call to prayer was a constant, like the sunrise. Prayers are called five times a day... such a comfort, as they never stopped...every day the same. When I came to live in England, I came to love the sound of the church bells in the same way, especially on a Sunday morning. Just like the town crier from days gone by they cried, "It's 12 o'clock and ALL IS WELL WITH THE WORLD." What a wonderful alternative!

61 Making the Best of a Bad Situation

I have four children. Each one of them is similar, yet different to the others, and to me, their motherboard (or Mother Ship, as my youngest calls me!) I was thinking of my Mother today. Time is unpredictable, how could it be so long since she died? How could it be that these last years have passed so quickly? I can remember her telling me that she had been blessed with an uncomplicated, happy childhood, with no great trauma.

"It's odd," she said, when talking about her childhood during the war, "I am ashamed to say that they were some of the happiest years of my life!"

What she meant was, it was exciting living in a small town far from London and far enough from Coventry to be safe from the bombing but near enough to experience American soldiers and all the fun that came with them. She had lots of freedom and she and her friends exploited it. Her Mother (my Grandmother) also had freedom. She got a job in a factory and enjoyed the social life and working to earn money. She was of an old generation and it was truly liberating. I was thinking about how my Mother, so full of life and mischievousness, ended up falling in love with an Arab student and living in Iraq in the 50s. She had a primitive life but was not alone. Other western women had also followed the same route, and they had a good social group. My Father was never going to be rich, and poverty followed her back here to England when we were exiled in 1960. She always said that she coped with everything flung at her because of the stability of her youth. But she had a fantastic attitude to life! It isn't just what you are faced with that challenges you, much depends on how you deal with it. My Mother was a very optimistic and solid person. I, on the other hand, don't mind a little melancholy; I am familiar with it. So we have choices, yes? But how we are made has a lot to do with attitude.

Harvest the fields of grain my son
Bring the fruits from the tree my daughter
Lay the feast upon the table my mother
Then bless this house my father
For all the abundance in our lives is the harvest of our
*   labors,*
But we are also the Alchemy of The Soul, and therefore the
*   unknown*
For I lived in a Circle all my life, my body curled around the
*   cord, spiraling towards the opening*
I yielded and I fought, my heart began to pound
The color rose in my skin and I reached for the light, though
*   my eyes were shut tight*
Birth came uninvited

62 Fear and Loathing

I did something today that I should have done some time ago. I went to a new dentist. I hate dentistry (not dentists) and suffer a lot of pain...three injections and still pain. My Grandmother always said she would prefer to have a baby than go to the dentist. Maybe that's why I 'podded' four at home, no painkillers, no problem, and yet dentistry terrifies me. Anyhow, this new dentist, he didn't know me nor I him. He was not aware that I was scared because my other dentist was not so great and I always had a lot of pain. So I was very defensive and honestly offensive. My first visit, not great: second visit, wow no pain! Third visit, I am a devotee. So I spoke to his wife in her hijab and apologized profusely for being so upset on the first two occasions. Her face lit up and her internal veil dropped. I felt so good seeing her smile. I told her that her husband was a wonderful dentist and that everyone in our community felt the same. "That means so much to us," she said. I felt tiny and humbled, because I felt happy and so did she. *Salam Alahkum.*

63 Death is Final

What a terrible shock it is to discover this. Someone very young died this weekend and it has affected us all. She was vibrant, inspiring and healthy. It was not an accident that killed her; it was her heart that gave up. If life is measured by breaths, not by years, then she had breathed her life.

64

Remember me as you would remember the snow
It is soft, yet cold, the sun may shine on me but I do not
*   melt as I drift*
I am made of many intricate patterns, designed to reflect
*   light*
I rest on the earth but am of the sky
Remember me like the snow, for I will return
Though I will not be the same

65 Step in the Right Direction, with Purpose

I told my child today that she is so negative about herself. I said to her, "You are capable of anything."

She said, "No, I'm not!"

The mind is a tool, not our master. Control the mind and we overcome the negative voice. Why is it we find we are happier listening to the negative and get annoyed at the suggestion of listening to the positive? Is it about failure? If we don't try we won't have to fail. But surely that is a failure in itself? I believe in purpose. We all have a purpose and it's a duty to find out what it is. The Jewish faith says it's God's will that we excel at the talents he gives us. It's a duty, a *dharma* to follow your talent. What a different attitude that is. It's good to be a success, but it's the way in which we conduct ourselves that counts. A fear of success has always interested me; it's much more a case of discovering what you are successful at.

People talk about being on a path and honestly...

— • • • —

I believe that finding your purpose is most likely to happen off the path.

— • • • —

66 Memory Boxes are Created by Each Event We Experience

It seems that recollecting a memory makes it clearer, more vivid and more understandable than in the moment we were living it. Our brain takes a million or more small frames of all we see every single day. We are often unaware of this until we recall those frames, and, amazingly, there they are. So, do we experience the present by reaching back into the past? Perhaps, and I don't see why that shouldn't be a valid way of seeing events. Like seeing the back of your head in your mirror, reflected by another mirror behind you.

67 Yogi Behaving Badly

I really do try to behave. I had a million little jobs to do today and a lot of intense work, too. Sitting in my local coffee shop with my Mac, I felt pretty relaxed and able to cope. I had taken the only clear space, a large coffee table with a small sofa and two chairs. As the place got busier, I had my head down. I like those times when the place is empty and I'm completely focused, then I suddenly get pulled out of my concentration and notice the place is full of people, noisy and lively. Anyway, I was behaving. A middle-aged couple began to hover around the table and I could see they were not sure whether to sit or not... so English. I made a gesture that they should sit. They spent the next 30 minutes talking about me. About my working on a Mac, about my iPhone, about my two phones, actually, as one is for personal use, the other work. I could feel the hairs on my neck go up and my eyes narrow. I really did try to behave. But, oh dear, I lost it. I didn't shout, I didn't become aggressive; I became snide! I hate that. I became sarcastic and suggested that rather than talk about me, they could consider leaving me in peace. I know they were shocked. And as I flew out of the place on my broomstick, I considered that maybe I had misread their comments and looks! Oh dear, I had been doing so well this week! I could only forgive myself and think, next time don't take anything personally, not anything!

68 A Brave Face

I heard the voice of the ego say slowly and carefully that it would help me to get through another day. "How?" I asked. By helping you see that being a pain and a grumpy old woman is perfectly acceptable, at your age, that is. I listened for a while, then decided to shut the door on the ego and smile very hard, till my lips curled up and the sun crept into my eyes and the dewy rose bloomed in my heart. It was hard work, but I managed it! Thank God!

69 Respect Without Question

Do you remember when you were little, how you would lie awake at nights considering what your parents had said and not really understanding it? My English Grandmother had some brilliantly confusing, mind-bendingly odd sayings. Such as "Bread and pull it." I can remember really trying to work out what 'bread and pull-it' was. Pull-it. Did she mean *poulet*, as in 'chicken'? I think I was nearly a hundred years old before I realized she meant 'bread and pull...it'...pull off a chunk of bread. She might also have meant, accept what you're given and be glad of it. Plus, it served the added purpose of shutting us up! Another was, "Nanna, how old are you?" (Very rude to ask in those days).

"I am as old as my eyes and a little older than my teeth."

I would just stand there with my eyes wide and my mouth drooling. Again, I did understand eventually; she was made at the same time as her eyes but her teeth arrived later. Discipline, in those days, was based around the concept that older was wiser. I never ever said, "What do you mean?" I just shut up. Brilliant.

As a mother of four (which I'm sure I've said many times, a bit like an overused excuse for being a little slower these days) I've learned that our children are sent to try us. If you ever thought that as you were older, you were therefore the wiser, then try bringing up a teenager in the 21st century - and think again. I now see my teenage daughter as a path to spiritual enlightenment! That's made me laugh, that's so good!

70 Perfect Mother/Father, Perfectly Ridiculous

I was the kind of mother who had a white set of clothes on, was never vomited on, never pooped on, had a clean house, sorted laundry, homemade bread, no car, read to all my children, gave them a hot breakfast every day (still do) and still managed to have all the other mums round for homemade cake, tea and lots of sympathy. Crikey! I must have been a big pain in their backsides! I would watch them struggle with children who screamed in the superstore, threw sandwiches at parties, cried till they got what they wanted (uh!) and pinched other kids when no one (but me) saw them. I honestly thought it must be the mother's fault. My kids were terrific when I took them out. They got on with everyone and were lovely. Then God said, "Ah! You need another child at forty!" OK, it's what I call another of God's jokes. Try it on for size, and spiritual (torture) growth. This child will knock all your sharp corners off, rub your face in the poop and then chuck you into a heap. Moral? Don't say anything that may draw attention to you and create a karmic response, especially at forty. I did consider writing that book...

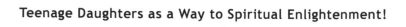

Teenage Daughters as a Way to Spiritual Enlightenment!

I think it may be worth saying at this point, that this beautiful, high-spirited, ferocious, creative child of mine has really helped me look at myself. I have learned to hold my tongue, breathe deeply, count to 101, grip the bannister, rather than throw myself over it, and to admire this young woman and her determination to be allowed to find herself, not with me but without me. Go girl!

71 Regret Nothing

As I write this I am in a bad place. I regret very little in life and I therefore feel sad that I lost my equilibrium and fell off my scales. I am in the dust, face down, and I deserve it. Honesty doesn't always pay, not when it comes down to someone else's feelings, and especially if that person is still really a struggling child. I forgive them, and then I try to forgive myself. Oh dear, I really should be alone right now; I am unable to show compassion to either others or myself.

•———— • • • ————•

But we all know it's easy to be a saint when you live in a room on your own.

•———— • • • ————•

72 Motherhood is the Point of no Return

B.C. 'Before Children', I could risk a lot. I was, of course, a child myself, with parents at the end of a phone or a signature lovingly scribed at the end of a letter. Once you have crossed the threshold of child-to-mother, the 'singles' door you once knew is closed.

It occurred to me that parenting was one of the hardest of all paths. Karma reaps havoc on us after we take on the responsibility of another human being. Every move we make is being observed and copied. 'What you sow, so shall you reap', is an apt statement once you have a child. All the imprints you make in this lifetime are deflected onwards and beyond in the personification of a small child, who copies and pastes all you taught again and again and again. So, when I woke up this morning, I scanned my mind quickly to try and remember why I had fallen asleep the night before in a hot sweat and with a jumpy heart. And I remembered that my son was struggling again with one of God's jokes. Yet again I stand confused while God laughs. So when I woke I had to pray and this is what came out.

"Dear God, I have to pray to you and ask that you give my son the gift of light. This is a purely selfish prayer because I cannot bear to see him falter. Give him light in his eyes that he may see where he is going. Give him light in his heart that he may feel where he is going. Give him light in his mind, that he may know what he is doing. Amen."

73 Saying Goodbye

I have held my Mother's ashes in a round, pink box since her cremation in 2009. Actually, her ashes are all over the place, not just in my pink box. I have sent some to my sister in Norway, and Mum is there, under a lilac tree. There are some in London, in her housing estate garden, under a bench dedicated to her, and in the Thames. There are more scattered outside her beloved Globe Theatre. She helped open it, a year after she was elected Mayor of Southwark, by reciting Shakespeare's 23rd Sonnet. We had her memorial there as it seemed apt, and the Globe directors offered us the space to remember her. My round, pink box came off the mantelpiece today. My son wanted to mark his 25th birthday by planting a palm tree at the bottom of the garden, in a very sunny spot. My Mother loved palms as they reminded her of Iraq. So there we are, me with my England shirt and he with his Leicester City one, sprinkling her ashes lovingly on the earth beneath the palm.

I have felt strange of late. I'm tired from working very hard but I can't say how I feel is because of that. I said goodbye to Mum today, and I know it. Am I tired of the process of saying goodbye? It has taken all my strength to hold back the act of letting go. I honestly thought I could see her by that tree, smiling as she always did, with a radiance that shone on us all. But I was deluded; she is quite simply, a ghost of a smile now.

Goodbye. I love you.

74

We consider ourselves Earth bound
Maybe in this human form we are
But our arms were once wings
Use them

75 Disappointment – A Measure of the Self

My child is disappointed that she got a 2.2 for her degree, when she felt she had worked hard enough for a 2.1. Bless her. No one is going to ask what grade her degree was. She travelled out to India after finishing a four year degree, and amazingly travelled the same journey her father and I travelled back in 1984. When she left, she took me with her, inside her. I felt I was experiencing India for the first time through her eyes. Interestingly, she is a lot more pragmatic than I am. She is already sick of roti and dal and could do with a pizza. I had to smile; I knew it. There was no point telling her she would get sick of the food, the sun, the toilet holes, the smell at times, but that she would be fine and carry on regardless. It's so like giving birth, every new experience. It can either feel out of control, in control, or in someone else's control, but just as quickly feel transcendental. I learned that each birth experience would be unique and could not be predicted. I learned to let go and let the wash, wash over me. It was horrendous but inevitable, as is much of life.

* * *

Horribly Wonderful.

* * *

76 An Email From a Happy Soul

Life does show different sides of itself when needs be. My daughter was ill for a few days, sick of roti for a couple more, but now is happier than she has ever been. Her ashram experience has released the knots and bumps of her body, soothed her exhausted soul after four years of study, and washed away the residue of make-up and girls' nights out, as well as allowed her to let her hair do its own 'thing'. Really happy she left her straighteners behind!

Learning about herself, her true self that is, is so exciting for her and for me. She was telling me about her chanting prayers and lecture times in the ashram. "I know what you're talking about Mum when you say Yoga changes you. Mum it reveals you, that's all!"

Honestly? My work is done. We spent a few moments chanting Jaya Ganesha together over the phone before she had to go and continue with her Karma Yoga. I know she had as big a smile on her face as was on mine.

Open your mind and so too will your heart, body and arms

open,
allowing all the wonders of life to run into them

77 Attachment

I find myself sitting in a familiar place, a favorite coffee shop. I drive to London each Sunday to train my teachers but I need that buffer between my children at home and my students (children) in the studio. The coffee is hitting the spot, but it's not left me feeling awful, just safe. Interesting, that our small daily rituals offer security and make us feel comfortable and comforted. I have just returned from an eight-day detox in a retreat in Spain, during which time I have had the privilege of teaching the art of meditation to complete Yoga novices. My method is to try to take the mystery, alienation, weirdness and fear out of meditating.

In one of my morning lectures, we began with understanding the mind's attachment to things, and especially familiar things, like a coffee, a tea, or a run in the morning. Some may say that out of those three things, one is positive. Which one? Running? Well, personally I don't see it like that; I see a ritual that makes us feel quiet inside, an opportunity to sit and contemplate or read. Cultures all around the world have a collective ritual such as Tai Chi, or Eurythmics, (Dalcroze Eurythmics, not to be confused with the musical group) an early morning run with friends or walking the dog. A dog will see his owner with the leash and think, 'walk time'. A child will see the rain outside and think, 'splashing in puddles time'. The mind associating thoughts or feelings with an action precipitates it becoming a ritual. We began thinking about these daily rituals when discussing meditation. The incense, the candle, a meditation shawl, all these items trigger the mind into saying, "It's meditation time." Working with this group gave me a great opportunity to break down the art of meditation into simple steps. I tried to make it easy, joyful and rewarding. I told my students they could do this right now, not tomorrow, but today. They began by sitting as straight as possible.

Step 1   The breath. Watch it by following it from nostril to belly and back, using the inner eye, not the outer eye.

Step 2   The breath. Watch it with full attention, slowing it down to watch more of its journey, to include the throat, chest and past the navel.

Step 3   Extend the spine more while sitting, allowing more breath to enter the body, watching it fill all the organs, muscles, cells and nerves.

Step 4   Imagine *Prana*, 'life force', 'Qui' or 'Chi', also winding its way into the body together with the breath. *Prana* expands us, allowing us to charge our batteries with subtle energy that illuminates, like the sun, every part of our physical and subtle body.

Step 5   Raise the eyes, with lids closed, towards the point between the eyebrows, the 'Third Eye', the pineal gland, where the windows of our inner world reside.

Step 6   I do nothing, say nothing and join them.

After around 15 minutes, I ask them to bring their awareness back to the body, to take a refreshing breath and to sigh. I ask them to flutter the eyes open, keeping their gaze low, and to allow the light to permeate the cells of the body. They 'wake up' gently.

"There you are," I say, "you have been meditating!"

The smiles of surprise, and some tears, too, are of genuine joy. So it's simple. Yes it is.

78 Money is Energy

I work very hard. I always have. I can say I've been working from a very young age and I've found it to be deeply satisfying. I enjoy earning money; there is a sense of achievement and some independence that goes with it. I'm older now...and wiser? I do see that you can't take anything with you when you 'pop your clogs', as I always say. It's an old expression that has a wonderful image with its horror. My children hate me saying it. I just laugh and say, "It's funny!" The idea of me in wrinkly black stockings, a headscarf, and my red clogs popping off my feet! It's hilariously funny to me!

It's a black comedy, and even more tragic when you realize that you leave the earth with nothing, just as you arrived.

We are all struggling financially. Even those with millions, because their lifestyle needs millions to fund it; it's all relative. Their million pound homes need that much to run and maintain them. How much harder it must be if you fall from so high up. While we, on the other hand, will only drop to our knees.

Karma Yoga is work for work's sake. It is doing a job and doing it well, with no hope or expectation of reward or remuneration. When we can achieve this, it brings total fulfillment and freedom. So accumulating wealth, and not using it for some good purpose, does seem a terrible waste.

As I've said previously, money is like any other energy; it needs to flow. The blood in our veins needs to move around the body in order to carry the oxygen and nutrients essential to our wellbeing to the various systems that make up our physical self. Money is no different. If it gets stuck in one place it makes us ill or kills us. Let the money flow. It keeps us part of the whole system, for when you give energy it flows back somehow, from right hand to left and back again. All energies are part of a flowing sequence of exchanges: not just the exchange of money but also the exchange of Love.

79 Mind Over Matter

The idea of mind over matter is a universal idiom for achieving what you want by controlling the matter, or body, by strengthening the mind. I can remember very clearly saying to an ex-lover, after a heated argument, that he had to go! I told him he must learn to use his mind to control his matter, rather than letting his matter control his mind! Not too proud of that now, but in essence what I was saying is that I was using my mind to control the matter of my emotion in our drama and so he didn't play a big part in my life anymore. I could have been more succinct about his role and said, "In the end I don't mind (what you do) and you don't matter!"

Our minds do help to control our feelings but just as easily, our feelings can control our mind. I watched an interesting documentary this evening, with David Malone, on what makes us human. It was quite brilliant, and for me this was due to the fact that he showed his feelings. Leonardo da Vinci made many discoveries about the human body, not least that the heart is beautiful, graceful and eloquent, because it does speak and is certainly not a machine. The idea of the heart being a mechanism came from the Victorian view of engineering and machinery as the most exquisite discovery of humans over nature. So the heart was presented to modern man not as poetry in motion but as machinery without emotion.

But how many times have you clutched your heart when in pain or in shock or when filled with compassion for another's suffering? The idea of being broken hearted is not a poetical myth but a real human expression of emotion. What amazes me the most is the idea that until science proves that our hearts respond physically to love, hurt, empathy, fear or joy, then this very real condition may continue to be ignored by health professionals when making their diagnosis. Poets have described the heart for centuries, because without acknowledging the heart there is no love, pain or fear; there is no human condition. *The Merchant of Venice* weighs the heart on his scales; a pound of flesh is what he wants. Why? Because everything a man or woman is, is of the heart.

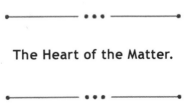

The Heart of the Matter.

I saw the symbol of the heart on the walls outside a temple in Egypt. It was in a set of hieroglyphics, telling the story of Isis and Osiris, their love for each other, and how she roamed the world, finding all the pieces of his body and putting them back together. The symbolism was so strong and clear – truly the heart is where the essence of being human resides, and when the heart becomes like stone it is because love, death or sorrow have become too painful to go on feeling. A heart of stone – A person with no feelings. My heartfelt thanks.

The hearth in a home, where the fire is, was called this because it was the 'Heart of the home'.

I love the English language. No wonder Shakespeare was English; he had the widest range of emotions at hand. English is my second language and because of this I see the depth of it. Downhearted, half-hearted, wholehearted. The matter of the heart is in us all.

80 Who is God? When will I know?

I had my usual, meaningful discussion with my brother today about understanding the Meaning of God, as opposed to the meaning of life. Did God create man, or did man create God?

I had been thinking about countries where disasters happen often, like tsunamis, earthquakes, fires, and the poverty that results from that. Yet these are the areas on our planet that have the strongest spiritual and religious beliefs. Life in these places can be so hard and these people desperately need some way to help them get through these terrible times. Prayer gives us strength to carry on when we don't think we can take another breath, much less another step.

So our conclusion was that man created God. This in no way makes God less or more, it is simply that God does exist now, and now we don't have to understand why. Though we do need to understand.

When things are terrifying, overwhelming, horrific, devastating, we drop to our knees, no matter what our beliefs and we pray. We pray for courage. Somehow that prayer is answered by way of finding something within us that enables us to take that next step, and the next, and the one after that: bravery born out of endurance, knowing that the sun will shine again: it is inevitable, as is recovery in some form or another. Even out of the most devastating circumstance, God willing, we live to see another day.

81

Love is the Angel of our Soul
Her wings beat like the heart, strong and constant
Her face is wise and compassionate and her eyes see all
*   there is to see*
Look upward and let the shade of her wings rest on your
*   face and rejoice in the moment*
You are Alive; you have life coursing through your veins
Walk out into the light and make a difference

82 Light and Shade

When dark clouds are inside your head and heart it's difficult to see how you move from there. The energy needed to make your feet move, or your arms, is often so hard come by that these simple tasks seem like the most difficult thing. Smiling seems impossible. Being positive is easily said, especially if you have never experienced depression or deep anxiety, but for anyone who has struggled in that dark space, it is, at that time, not possible. I found a book, years ago, when I thought I had to let go of my life; it was too painful and useless to fight anymore. I was buried deep within my dark place and no one would ever find me. Cheri Huber's book *Depression as a way to Spiritual Growth* jumped off a shelf into my hands. The message was clear, like all things we need to deal with or overcome, don't fight, surrender. Be in the pain, know where it sits, accept it and embrace it. Notice the breath and the parts of the body the pain moves to. I worked on a page each day, practicing not doing, accepting the terrible place I was in. No aims, no goals, no expectations. For me, it worked. I see the dark clouds still now and then on the horizon but the difference is, I see them, therefore I am acknowledging that they are still part of who I am. Life is as painful as it is glorious. Sun and Moon, light and shade, all are aspects of the same life, and faces of the same God.

83

I am the doer, the one who makes things happen
I am the reflection of God's gift of hope
In that moment of self-doubt I stand still and allow strength
*   to pour into me, because I can*

84 Sacrifice and Surrender

There is an Indian saying that goes like this:

> "When you decide to be a parent, you treat your child from birth to five as a God, from six to thirteen as your servant, and thereafter as your equal."
> *Anon*

I used to breast-feed my children all through the night. Feeding them myself was such a rewarding experience. With my first child I used to watch the clock, twenty minutes right breast, next feed, twenty minutes left breast. I began to realize that my child fed every forty minutes through the night and was ready for a good sleep by ten in the morning. That night I decided to get rid of the clock and surrender to the fact that I would rarely have time to myself, and if I did, it would be a bonus, not an expectation. I was so free after that and settled into feeding and giving and loving and being there for the rest of my life.

85 Make Time

And your friend did 103 things in the same day. She was in 'the zone' as they say, on a concentrated, focused rhythm. A bit like writing, some days it flows so your pen can hardly keep up, while other days the process drags endlessly and the mind is muddled.

So it's interesting when you meditate, because you are in both those spaces. Time stands still, time flies, time is endless, time is nothing.

"Make time," I say to my children, when they tell me they don't have any. It's not impossible; it's a skill.

Slow down the breathing, the in and the out, really slow, so you slow down. Breath and action, action and breath live side by side, interdependent. The accident you had when everything went into slow motion? You could see, hear and remember every minute detail. That is something we can learn to do. We may discover ourselves that time can only be measured by its content. You may have had a day that seemed agonizingly long. The clock seemed to be standing still, and yet your best friend said it flew by. The fact is, though, that you did little and she achieved a lot. When the mind is flitting about like a butterfly, it never has long enough to achieve its potential.

———— • • • ————

"It's all about the timing," said the little girl.
"When I jump and when I land. There is no point jumping sooner or later."
"It's a game of time and space," answered the clock.
"Ah yes," agreed the girl, "time and pace."

———— • • • ————

86 Respecting your Child's Path – Protecting Siddartha

Siddartha was the Buddha's name in 'real' life. His parents spent their time protecting him from the pain, squalor, disease, putrid smells and ageing of humanity. They never allowed him outside the high-walled boundary of the palace. His life was joyful, happy, I imagine, an idyllic childhood. As a parent we do try to protect our children from pain and suffering, it's natural to do so. In Siddhartha's case, he was like every other child; he needed to be curious, to rebel, to make his own way in life through exerting his personality and spirit. So he climbed the forbidden wall to enter the city outside his own realm of reality, his life. He experienced emotions (I imagine) that were uncomfortable. Smells of human and animal waste, of rotting food, and he witnessed something very frightening: old age. He was devastated, shocked, overwhelmed by feelings he had not experienced before, and it was this first rebellious journey outside his familiar, beautiful world that prompted his determination to help humans overcome the depths of emotion that allowed the mind to become discouraged, afraid, confused and depressed, and, ultimately, to help them overcome the fear of death.

Now, I have studied many philosophers and all have something to offer us. As a parent, I felt it was important that children were allowed to see death as a natural part of life. When my Father died, my children were still young but they were involved with the process of saying goodbye and letting my Father, their Grandfather, leave our lives with respect and love. They all put little notes, and things they thought he would like to take with him, into the coffin. This was not unlike the Egyptians, who would equip their deceased with what they thought they would need for their journey into the next life (afterlife). My Father died suddenly and I was not there to witness it. I was so broken; I thought I would never get over losing him. It took three years to be able to think of him without crying. His funeral was on a wonderful sunny day and there were very many people, some of whom I had never met. I have memories and photos of that day and think of it as a really 'good' day.

When my Mother was diagnosed with cancer, I let out a scream I didn't recognize as my voice. It came from a place I could hardly remember was me. Her death was the most horrific death I could imagine. She died in pain, anger and desperation, and ultimately, she was broken hearted. She loved life, and she never thought about death. Interestingly, she had not witnessed her own Mother's death from cancer, as she lived a long way away. I'm glad she didn't see her because she would never have been able to shake the devil from her back. My memories of Mum's death simply haunt me. The specter of her dying comes to me in glimpses out of the shadows, in moments of action or inaction. Her bodiless form lingers like a perfume on a good day, like a ghost on a bad one. My conclusion is that maybe we should keep the horrors of life and death away from our children. Maybe forcing radical ideas of nature onto them is not the best thing for their young minds. I'm thinking twice about whether I did the right thing. What I do know is that as a parent, no matter what I do, I will be wrong. My youngest daughter fought to be at her other Grandfather's funeral. In the north-east, it's not normal to allow children to a funeral but my child felt she was being pushed out and excluded, so she came, with my blessing. Would I have done it differently? I don't think so. In the end a child must be allowed to find out who they are by the measure of strength they find in the crisis of a moment.

87 How to Loosen the Hold

Letting something lose its grip on you is very hard if what you're required to let go of is love. I loved my parents as my 'parents', though at times it was tough, but I also loved them as individuals. I cleared their homes after they died. I realized that holding onto them had been harder than letting go.

88

As I stand here, alone, I am holding onto my memories like
a ribbon entwined around my body
I need to unravel, to turn around and unwind, to allow my

body to discover its freedom
I am free of pain, of loss and of my parents now
I embrace my new role in life and begin to weave my own
    ribbons
My children will hold them and one day do as I am doing,
    let go

89 Counting Out Our Blessings

My Mother would always remind us, "There is always someone worse off than you."

I didn't really understand what she meant because, when I was small, I thought that we all had the same life. It wasn't until I went to school that I began to realize that we weren't all the same when it came to our houses and what we had in them, or our clothes and where they came from, or the food we ate and where we bought it. We were often in abject poverty but I didn't see this either till I met people who had chocolate any day, not just Christmas Day: who had a biscuit tin on the side everyday, not just Fridays and whose parents never said, "I love you".

I heard a lovely discussion about the subject of what you have or don't have and the desire for more.

This old Indian gentleman said, "We are happy to be alive and each day we wake up is a blessing. You in the west, you measure your happiness by the things you own and that is why you are never happy, because you cannot own everything."

If you have never been to India then this may be hard to grasp, but poverty is a better state than most in the urban life of Indians. Often they own nothing but what they stand up in, and though their lives may seem wretched by our own standards, they will always tell you there is someone worse off than them.

When circles begin to meet, touching end to end and the earth's spirals unwind
Then time becomes a loosened knot and life a lotus stem

90 Random Meetings

How is it that people meet like a clash of marbles rolling in a playground? Some without awareness and others with an eye for a chance to collide and crack open. Random meetings are never random but a game set against the backdrop of an emotion or commotion. From chaos comes calm and then rest, as the marbles continue to roll away to cross another's path.

Once upon a time, when all beings knew no bounds and the sky had no eye for a storm, the three Graces lighted upon the Earth, touching only with the lightest of touches. 'Divine Understanding', her face enraptured with awe, 'Spirited Heart', with eyes of courage glowing, and the brother, the 'Shield Bearer', who, with an arm stronger than the wind, encircled his sisters. Their wings, held together with home and compassion, protected the beings on Earth with a silent strength known only by the one consciousness. Life was as it always was and life gave thanks to all the beings breathing life.

91

Sleep is a ghost of Rest
It neither lets you close your mind, nor your fears
Dreams play out with such passion, sharpness and clarity of feeling
But the lens of sleep is often narrow, faded
With spaces where your hopes will fill the void
The night's waking is a lurch, a shunted movement

A second of not-remembering
Better to rest with conscious thought
The breath leading the mind
The mind releasing life's scribbles left on the bones
The only way to realize your dream is to wake up!

92 A New Dance

It's New Year. There is a knock at my door. I open it to a young person, small, rounded and pale. She is Indian but was born here, so her English is perfect. She wants to buy a DVD from me. We stand awkwardly on the threshold and I sense a reluctance to leave. "What else is it you need?" I ask. She tells me that a gym has told her she needs to lose weight, but she is unable to focus or concentrate on anything. I don't think she needs to lose weight; she needs help with concentration. I have a very strong feeling that there is something that is the root cause of her anxiety. I gently suggest there might be one thing in her life that is tipping her over; it may be a small thing, I tell her, but none the less important. She stands still, looking at me as though she has just woken up. "My mother," she admits. Ah! It becomes obvious I cannot keep her on the doorstep. I ask her to come in and sit down.

Her story is short and clear. She is the only daughter, in a family of three children, still unmarried and at home. She is 31. She shakes like a little mouse; if she was a mouse she would have put her little paws in front of her face and wept. I am a mother. I had to take her in. I give her a simple mantra, an idea, a way of helping her that may be, in essence, similar to her prayers to God. "I love my mother, but I cannot live with her." Her face opens and I see a horizon in her eyes - hope.

"I will remember that for the rest of my life," she says.

We sit and talk about the practical steps she can take to

move out and to start living a grown up life...her life, not her mother's. She had become so battered spiritually that she lived in her mother's shadow. I remind her of the concept of *Ahimsa*, on which Hinduism is based, on non-violence in word, thought or deed. I tell her that as long as she kept her integrity she must see her actions as survival, and actually, that her mother's life was just that...her mother's story.

93

Maturity has that essence of knowing when to stay and when to leave
The understanding that happiness is a sprinkling of love, not an avalanche

94 Divine Introspection

Divine Introspection
I catch a glimpse of the shadow
that falls upon my hands
I watch, my fingers uncurled
as the shadow-play begins
Divine Incubation
My body is like a spacesuit
I orbit around my Mother's navel
I am weightless
I am Alice in Wonderland
Falling like a pack of wolves
Touching the Earth, softly
I speak with Divine Inflection
Om Om Om Om Om Om Om Om

Sitting talking to my teachers today, I pointed out that learning on such a course was much more about their use of Yoga in their lives than about the people that they may meet on the way. We laughed as I suggested that if they forgot what to do next they could put their students in a seated pose, they could Om and, with eyes closed, breathe. I told them that as they sat there they could silently act out a scene from Laurel & Hardy: pulling their hair out to help them remember. This genuine truth from my 37 years' experience made them laugh a lot! But I also told them that my teaching had got me through some of the worst of times and how, while they sat silently, eyes closed, breathing, I was crying, or holding on to the edge of the cliff top, my fingers bleeding because of the awful time I was going through. Teaching is a lifeline, 90 minutes of forgetting, an hour and a half of absorption into practice and gifting. There was a room of incredulous faces looking at me and thinking, 'I didn't expect that,' but there was also relief that perfection was not what teaching or Yoga was about, but rather it was about finding a way to deal with some of the harshest and cruelest of God's jokes.

95 Remember to Forget

Thinking about people you loved who are now dead, gone to 'somewhere over the rainbow', can bring up so many floating memories and images that our body, and especially our heart, starts to respond to them. Alzheimer's disease, striking the older person, is only full of suffering for us who are seemingly forgotten. Recognizing that your dear friend, mother, father is flitting in and out of 'real time', the 'moment', then back to memory time, allows us to see that their pain increases when we are forgotten and show it. Once Alzheimer's takes over fully, as long as there are no triggers for memory recall, then they become free. If we can only believe in this very moment, whatever the experience, physical pain, mental pain or emotional pain will pass.

Pain is very real and when inflicted by someone significant in our lives, who is also cruel, then it can destroy us, tearing apart the very fabric that makes us who we are. But if we have choices in other ways, such as suffering being optional, then let's opt not to suffer and to just recognize we have time to be the better person we strive to be. I am, in essence, whole, and I allow myself to stop and un-do.

96

Learning to be alone rather than suffering in lone-liness
Loneliness is about the ego's hold on our mind-heart
Alone is a chance to be quiet
Change loneliness to Aloneness and connect that feeling to
*   God*
All-one-ness

97 Fear is Real

I read a lot, a mixture of authors, genres and styles, from modern to ancient. I read many spiritual books. Fear is something that is talked about a lot. Feel the fear etc. etc. ...

But today I am facing a very real fear, not an abstract one, not one that is faceless and arises through panic or depression. It came to mind that when a prisoner is faced with judgment, when he knows he is innocent, or a young person knows their abuser is coming, that they are the ones facing their fears, because that fear is not imagined, it's not about the past or the future but about the now. This is when I want to get hold of the authors of those books who say 'face your fear, be in the moment' and scream at them that, "Fear for some is REAL and it's here in REAL TIME. So don't delude yourself for God's Sake!"

Yes, I feel so strongly that I cannot, will not, should not ever assume for a moment that the fear someone is experiencing is not every bit as real in the past, future or PRESENT. Respect the ones who fear their reality, they are in the here and NOW!

98 Stay Real

Because I practice Yoga, people ask me if I ever get angry, do I swear, have I done anything to be ashamed of? I always answer, "Well of course I have, and still do, but just imagine how much worse it would be if I didn't practice Yoga!"

Never pretend to be anything other than who you really are. Admit to 'not knowing'; admit that you are human and trying to live a good life. Jesus, when he went into the wilderness and the devil sat with him, admitted he could do no more, could not save the world. The Devil said, "Yeah, leave them, they will be OK without you." It was then that Jesus, as a human being, realized he could never leave a soul to suffer and that his duty was to show compassion. Be human and place your feet upon the footsteps of God and let him make your burden lighter.

Draw back the curtain of illusion
Behind the anger and the pain is a lesson to be learned
Remind yourself you are a reflection and that when you loved
You looked into the face of God

99 One Name for God

"Awareness.
One name for God."
-*Ram Dass*

———— • • • ————

You cannot 'do' Awareness.
You can only 'BE' Awareness.
Our face is a reflection of the God within us.
We need to 'see' to be 'aware' of 'our' God.

———— • • • ————

100 Silence that Surpasses All Understanding

Ridiculous as it might seem, for one who practices Yoga and meditation, all I wanted today was silence. Surely I always have it? No, not profound silence: the sound so powerful it's noisy – or the sound that is so still. I was in the Greek island of Lesbos, training and teaching over a period of six summers. On a rare day off I got into my tiny hire car with three close friends and we proceeded to make an almost second and third trip around the island. The roads there are often scarily non-existent and crumbly along the mountain's cliff edge. I drove higher, off the main road, towards a working monastery of the Greek Orthodox faith. It had a high, arched entrance, a few lions roaring on the precipice, and the monks' ghostly shadows moving about. They seemed to have many stray cats happily lying in the sun around the inner courtyard, where there were strong balconies with rugs over them and a well for fresh water. Plants and pots decorated the steps and well-side. In that inner courtyard was their church. It was very hot and the church was welcomingly cool. As I stepped from outer to inner, the silence was so thick that my heart held its beat, as if it was too noisy.

I love monasteries, convents and churches and I have seen many in the world that are majestic in their architecture. This one was simple but ornate, a miniature cathedral. But its silence was a silence created over many hundreds of years. Layer upon layer of silence and focused thought on God, prayer and stillness. My friends stood in that silence and I can only describe it as ether filled with prayer. As I reached my hand out into its space I could see the silence move before me, my hand leaving its prints there.

I thought I had experienced silence in the Himalayas, The Rocky Mountains, Mount Kailash in Southern India, but no, this was SILENCE beyond all understanding.

How blessed was I. Once tasted never forgotten.

101 A Silent Day

A silent day for me, needed to hear my thoughts, taking time to breathe and spend time letting my inner voice be heard. I took a walk in the gentle snow, not the settling kind but the snow that is rain in slow, visible motion.

I looked up, rather than down, and noticed my thoughts as they stayed with me, noticing my child inside and behind me, seeing through my eyes.

I needed answers and direction, so I asked for just that.

Guide me without judgment
Lead me without regret
Reveal my path under my feet and, as I walk
Let me see my steps in that gentle snow

Those behind and those in front, and those I cannot see

102 Fall Down and Out

I am back in a troubled place and, yes, I know I talk about this a lot, but this is a part of my life and a part I must live with.

I have struggled with health issues these last two years, it took that long to find out why I wanted to lie down on the sofa with a blanket by 3.30 in the afternoon. I had a tumor on my parathyroid gland, behind the thyroid. It was benign but without its removal I would have ended up with osteoporosis. This gland regulates the calcium the body produces and when it overworks it leeches the calcium from the bones, so when I broke my wrist in two places in 2014 alarm bells went off. It caused depression, too, but I have that anyway so I didn't notice!

The night I broke my wrist, I remember the moment I lost my attention and tripped. Was it a cry for help? I was exhausted. It's no excuse, but I remember 'cloudily' that a thought drifted across my mind 'I am so tired', and that was the moment I fell. It was an awkward fall that twisted my arm and wrist right around so I landed on the right side of my face, the arm cushioning the blow. My wrist, at a distorted and grotesque angle, took the fall. I'm not certain whether the 'bang' of the break was real or in my head but it was loud, like a gunshot.

• • •

I was down and I was out.

• • •

103

I find out about the truth
My fingertips were white with holding on
Toes scratching the edge of the cliff
Slower and slower my mind thinks
Each second a day, every thought a year
Heart stops in motion
Blood moves fast but invisibly
Am I dying?
Am I living?
I am both here and there now
Will I fall between the cracks, or will I let myself fall?
God is there only to watch, to forgive no matter the choice
Or did God let me go?

104 Build a Palace

I am the pillar and post of my children's lives. I hold up the ceiling and keep the doors open. I have no 'soft place' to fall. It's a hard, gravelly surface that is there to hold me, and though it was painful that winter night, I fell and broke myself. I have searched and struggled with my soul to agree on the reason it happened. It didn't make my life easier: in fact, it continues to be a challenge. I could not practice that which had saved me all those years ago and was my continual savior throughout my life: my own personal, physical Yoga each day.

I am a brutally honest person and I know for a fact that I could find no other rational or legitimate way to opt out of my work for a while. That sounds desperate and I think it was.

———— • • • ————

Why do we engineer disasters when we could be
building palaces?

———— • • • ————

105 Judge Not Thyself

I believe in the Voice of Reason. My health is under attack right
now and I am not used to it. I'm the one who watches as others
find themselves in 'dis-ease'. Is this arrogance that I'm seeing
in myself? If it is, I don't like it.

It occurred to me at this low point, that if my heart is down
then I'm undermining my own health and that I need to stop
deluding myself and accept that I have issues I must resolve.

So I sat myself down and closed my eyes. It's easy to hide
from yourself when you're busy, but stopping still and 'noticing'
is one way of removing the mask you wear each day. I simply
slowed down long enough to become aware of the thoughts
floating to the surface. I needed to stay on the subject of my
health and my heart, so pushed away any other thoughts that
wanted to make themselves known.

I found myself accessing images, pictures of past events,
such as my Mother's dying and death. Interesting how sharp
those recollections were, considering they were back in 2009.
They seemed to be on a loop, first her alive, then telling me she
had cancer, then the hospital appointments, the wheelchair, the
smell of chemotherapy, her denial and anger at my suggesting
we talk about what she wanted after her death and her never
saying goodbye to me.

I had so much guilt around my emotions here, stemming
from such minute details such as not letting her help me in

the kitchen when she visited me at weekends. I thought I was spoiling her by letting her rest, now I see that she just wanted to be with me.

Even now I feel sick thinking about how she might have felt rejected.

Mum I am so sorry...If only I had taken more time to be 'with you' and not just 'there for you'.

I've been punishing my heart and now it's wounded because of my own self-judgment. I must try to remember that my Mother was loved, deeply loved and she loved me.

Dear Ones,
What has gone before is in the past and never to be revisited. Letting go of the guilt and the sorrow, you are left with love and all that it represents.
Judge not others but just as imperative, judge not your-self.

106 Worry Not

I decided to access the Rose Alchemy cards I use to steady me. These are based around the essence of the rose and its unique quality.

It's not a new concept. The rose and its relationship to the heart are found in Christian and Islamic art and have been symbols of love and compassion for many thousands of years.

I chose three cards: past, present and future. Each card has a photo image of a rose that is different in color and species and therefore its qualities and resonances are also individual. Drawing a particular card speaks to the user with that rose's own message. As in most 'divination' cards, you can ask a specific question or allow your intuition to do the asking without conscious application. I chose to do that.

I lay my three cards face down in the order of past, present and future.

Card one, the past, was a vibrant yellow rose that I could smell and sense without any difficulty. Its message was very clear indeed! Joy! It read as, 'What has happened that stopped you playing? What do you do for fun'? This hit me hard but it stirred my sense of humor, too. I had lost my mojo, my passion for living. I needed to 'lighten up'!

Card two, the present, was a red rose, so dark I wanted to fall into its velvet folds. This card suggested I was working very hard, as usual, on preserving the status quo. As a single mother of four, my response was audible! Well, of course, what else should I be doing? But was I measuring myself by my work and not by my essence, the real me? It also occurred to me that I spent a lot of time analyzing my own purpose and that I could be just 'in the work' and not 'of the work'. Um, maybe that was what the card was trying to tell me!

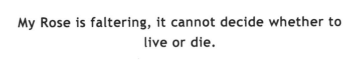

My Rose is faltering, it cannot decide whether to live or die.

Card three, the future, was a rose another shade of red, a softer shade, with dew on its petals. I felt I had been drawn into its perfume, so like my meditation practices that sometimes take me into the edges of the 'City of Light', to a place of Bliss. The message here was to stop worrying about the greater plan. We need only be aware of the steps that take us towards it.

I couldn't believe I had to be told this: after all, it's what I teach on a daily basis!

Smacked fingers for me then...seemingly all of us need to be constantly reminded to practice that vital message in all that we think, in what we say and how we act.

A Message to Me
I close my eyes to stop it
No more of others' pain
I unzip my leaden body
I jump out and flutter
Stay smiling my true love
No more of others' pain you bear
You are your own true love, my dear

107 Soul Purpose

I read a lot about women saints, modern day Buddhist nuns and spiritual women scientists. The echoes through all of these women's lives have been hard work, discipline and daily endeavor, day in, day out, year after year.

If we decide to dedicate ourselves to improving our lives, to making our sojourn on this Earth purposeful and happier, then we need to work at it. How many times have we promised ourselves that tomorrow we are going to get up and practice our meditation, our Yoga, start to take a daily jog around the park or begin that project?

We are the Great Procrastinators!

The one thing we humans battle with the most is laziness. Harsh words? No, I don't think so, because each time you give in to your mind when it tells you - it's OK, don't get up early, give yourself a treat and lie in - you become weaker. Every time you push one more step, one more breath, one more Sun

Salutation, one more minute of meditation, you get stronger.

Really, what is the point of aspiring to a better life if you don't work at it? If you've given up your life to a faith, then why not trust it? You can't have it all if you don't know what you want. They say it is a sin to have knowledge (knowing how to improve your life) and then not to use it and not to hand it on...but of course, this is a big responsibility and maybe you feel you just can't make that extra effort.

There you go again, your mind getting the better of you!

Fight the desire to give in, fight the urge to ignore your intuition, fight for your faith...your mind will always win if you don't get in the habit of doing the right thing...every day, and in every way.

Let your Soul's Purpose take the lead and hand over to the Divine, after all, it's what you wish for, hope for and pray for.

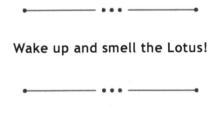

Wake up and smell the Lotus!

108

I thought I saw a rainbow flash past my eyes as the grey skies drove the wind and rain into my face.

The reflections of the rainbow left some faint remains of color on the dark stone of the temple and I knew then, that I had seen God playing in the rain.

So Where am I Now?

If only I had known that the ground was soft after the rain and hard after the drought.

Maybe then I would not have stumbled so often and lost my way.

So I looked out for the signs in the sky, like the Eagle and the Dove.

Each one of them had a Spirit that I felt I could trust in and follow.

They led me to the Top of the Mountain and there I found the Healer who asked me to sit and wait a while.

I waited One Hundred and Eight Years in Ignorance, till I understood; The Healer was I.

Note to Reader

Thank you for reading *108 Steps to God*. It takes a moment of inspiration or more often, desperation, to reach out for help. In whatever form that help comes, trusting your own instincts is a vital step in acquiring the answer.

If you have a few moments, please feel free to add your review of the book at your favorite online site. Also, if you would like to read my other books, please visit my website www.sun-power-yoga.co.uk for news, recent blog posts and to sign up for my newsletter.

Anne-Marie

Suggested reading

Anne-Marie Newland	*Sun Power Yoga SHALA*
Sister Wendy (Wendy Beckett):	*Meditations on Joy*
	Joy Lasts on the Spiritual in art
	Book of Meditations
	Sister Wendy on Prayer
	Check out her BBC documentaries.
Hildegard of Bingen:	*Book of Divine Works: With Letters and Songs*
Saint Theresa of Lisieux:	*Story of the Soul*
Tenzin Palmo:	*Cave in the Snow*
A film by Jody Kemmerer:	Sky Dancer: A Teacher of Timeless Wisdom (A film about the daily life and teachings of one of Tibetan Buddhism's great female masters, Khandroma Kunzang Wangmo.)
Keith Dowman:	*Sky Dancer: The Secret Life and Songs of the Lady Yeshe Tsogyel*

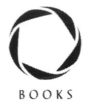

BOOKS

O-BOOKS

SPIRITUALITY

O is a symbol of the world, of oneness and unity; this eye represents knowledge and insight. We publish titles on general spirituality and living a spiritual life. We aim to inform and help you on your own journey in this life.
If you have enjoyed this book, why not tell other readers by posting a review on your preferred book site? Recent bestsellers from O-Books are:

Heart of Tantric Sex
Diana Richardson
Revealing Eastern secrets of deep love and intimacy to Western couples.
Paperback: 978-1-90381-637-0 ebook: 978-1-84694-637-0

Crystal Prescriptions
The A-Z guide to over 1,200 symptoms and their healing crystals
Judy Hall
The first in the popular series of six books, this handy little guide is packed as tight as a pill-bottle with crystal remedies for ailments.
Paperback: 978-1-90504-740-6 ebook: 978-1-84694-629-5

The 7 Myths about Love...Actually!
The journey from your HEAD to the HEART of your SOUL
Mike George
Smashes all the myths about LOVE.
Paperback: 978-1-84694-288-4 ebook: 978-1-84694-682-0

The Holy Spirit's Interpretation of the New Testament
A course in Understanding and Acceptance
Regina Dawn Akers
Following on from the strength of *A Course In Miracles*, NTI
teaches us how to experience the love and oneness of God.
Paperback: 978-1-84694-085-9 ebook: 978-1-78099-083-5

The Message of A Course In Miracles
A translation of the text in plain language
Elizabeth A. Cronkhite
A translation of *A Course in Miracles* into plain, everyday
language for anyone seeking inner peace. The companion
volume, *Practicing A Course In Miracles*, offers practical lessons
and mentoring.
Paperback: 978-1-84694-319-5 ebook: 978-1-84694-642-4

Thinker's Guide to God
Peter Vardy
An introduction to key issues in the philosophy of religion.
Paperback: 978-1-90381-622-6

Your Simple Path
Find happiness in every step
Ian Tucker
A guide to helping us reconnect with what is really important in
our lives.
Paperback: 978-1-78279-349-6 ebook: 978-1-78279-348-9

365 Days of Wisdom
Daily Messages To Inspire You Through The Year
Dadi Janki
Daily messages which cool the mind, warm the heart and guide
you along your journey.
Paperback: 978-1-84694-863-3 ebook: 978-1-84694-864-0

Body of Wisdom
Women's Spiritual Power and How it Serves
Hilary Hart
Bringing together the dreams and experiences of women across
the world with today's most visionary spiritual teachers.
Paperback: 978-1-78099-696-7 ebook: 978-1-78099-695-0

Practicing A Course In Miracles
A Translation of the Workbook in Plain Language and With
Mentoring Notes
Elizabeth A. Cronkhite
The practical second and third volumes of The Plain-Language
A Course In Miracles.
Paperback: 978-1-84694-403-1 ebook: 978-1-78099-072-9

Readers of ebooks can buy or view any of these bestsellers by
clicking on the live link in the title. Most titles are published
in paperback and as an ebook. Paperbacks are available in
traditional bookshops. Both print and ebook formats are
available online.
Find more titles and sign up to our readers' newsletter at
http://www.johnhuntpublishing.com/mind-body-spirit
Follow us on Facebook at https://www.facebook.com/OBooks/
and Twitter at https://twitter.com/obooks